Understanding 25 RARE DISEASES – LUNG

Chapter 1 – LAM - "Lymphangioleiomyomatosis"
Chapter 2 – PCD - "Primary Ciliary Dyskinesia"
Chapter 3 – PAP - "Pulmonary Alveolar Proteinosis"
Chapter 4 – PAH - "Pulmonary Artery Hypertension"
Chapter 5 – LCH - "Langerhans Cell Histiocytosis"
Chapter 6 – BOOP - "Bronchiolitis Obliterans Organizing Pneumonia"
Chapter 7 – Sarcoidosis
Chapter 8 – IPF - "Idiopathic Pulmonary Fibrosis"
Chapter 9 – AATD – "Alpha-1 Antitrypsin Deficiency"
Chapter 10 – DAH "Diffuse Alveolar Hemorrhage"
Chapter 11 – ILD - "Interstitial Lung Disease"
Chapter 12 – PLCH - "Pulmonary Langerhans Cell Histiocytosis
Chapter 13 – Amyloidosis
Chapter 14 – PF + BMF -"Pulmonary Fibrosis with Bone Marrow Failure"
Chapter 15 – WG + PA - "Wegener's Granulomatosis with Polyangiitis"
Chapter 16 – GP – "Goodpasture's Syndrome"
Chapter 17 – COP - "Cryptogenic Organizing Pneumonia"
Chapter 18 – Actinomycosis
Chapter 19 – HP - "Hypersensitivity Pneumonitis"
Chapter 20 – EG - "Eosinophilic Granuloma"
Chapter 21 – Berylliosis
Chapter 22 – PAM - "Pulmonary Alveolar Microlithiasis"
Chapter 23 – LIP - "Lymphocytic Interstitial Pneumonia"
Chapter 24 – Lymphocytic Bronchiolitis
Chapter 25 – DIP - "Desquamative Interstitial Pneumonia"

"Lymphangioleiomyomatosis - LAM" - A Comprehensive Understanding

Subtitle: An Insight into Etiology, Clinical Symptomology, Radiological Evaluation, Management, and Treatment of Lymphangioleiomyomatosis

Incidence: 3-5 / million
M/F: Almost entirely in Female

Introduction:

Lymphangioleiomyomatosis (LAM) is an uncommon yet significant disease that strikes primarily during the prime years of womanhood. This progressive, widespread condition exhibits its influence through a series of physiological abnormalities, most crucially through an erratic multiplication of smooth muscle-like cells.

This rapid proliferation contributes to an inevitable destruction of lung tissue, forming numerous cysts that drastically impair lung function. In addition, LAM is also known to cause deformations in lymphatic systems and kidneys, thereby investigating a broader anatomical impact than primarily anticipated.

However, the multi-faceted nature of LAM often results in it remaining unnoticed or inaccurately understood within the medical fraternity. This ambiguity stems from the overarching symptoms that closely mimic several other respiratory and renal diseases, coupled with its scarcity which limits exposure and hence, comprehensive understanding.

Unfortunately, such underdiagnosis or misinterpretation carries the potential for severe repercussions, primarily through delayed interventions and management strategies that could otherwise significantly enhance the quality of life and lifespan of the affected individuals (Johnson & Taveira-DaSilva, 2016).

Moreover, unravelling the intricacies of LAM necessitates in-depth scientific exploration into its etiology and clinical symptomology. Comprehending the causes and progression of the disease will arm researchers and healthcare professionals with valuable insights, propelling accurate diagnosis, effective disease management, and progressive treatment modules.

Likewise, a comprehensive radiological assessment might prove instrumental in unriddling LAM's extensive impact on the intricate network of the lungs, lymph, and kidneys.

Ultimately, as the medical and scientific communities delve deeper into the realm of LAM, the hope remains to demystify its complexities and thereby further the prospects of efficient management and treatment. Hence, enabling a gateway to healthier, fulfilled lives for those who face the tribulations of Lymphangioleiomyomatosis.

Etiology and Epidemiology:

The exact etiology of LAM is not entirely understood. It is proposed to be of neoplastic origin with a growth advantage for LAM cells. This disease is classified into two types: sporadic (S-LAM) and associated with tuberous sclerosis complex (TSC-LAM). S-LAM is not associated with any inherited genetic conditions, and TSC-LAM is associated with inherited mutations in the TSC1 or TSC2 genes involved in inhibiting cell growth and division (Taveira-DaSilva et al., 2015). The epidemiological prevalence of LAM varies from 1.3 to 7.7 per million women in the general population.

Clinical Symptoms:

Clinical presentation varies based on the extent of lung involvement and presence of abdominal complications like renal angiomyolipomas and lymphatic tumors. The common clinical symptoms of LAM range from an asymptomatic presentation to mild breathlessness, and progressively severe dyspnea on exertion, chylus accumulations (chylothorax, chylopericardium, chylous ascites), recurrent spontaneous pneumothorax, chest pain, and occasional hemoptysis. Symptoms related to TSC such as seizures, mental retardation, and skin abnormalities may be present in TSC-LAM patients (Amitani et al., 1992).

Radiological Evaluation:

High-resolution computed tomography (HRCT) is recommended for the radiological evaluation of LAM due to its high sensitivity and specificity. A typical HRCT presentation includes thin-walled, round, well-defined uniform cysts scattered diffusely throughout normal lung parenchyma. In advanced stages, the dense cystic pattern endows a characteristic "honeycomb" appearance (Crausman et al., 1996).

Treatment/Management:

The management approach for LAM emphasizes slowing disease progression, managing complications, and improving the quality of life. Pharmacotherapy with mTOR inhibitors such as Sirolimus or Everolimus are recommended, decreasing the size of chylous effusions and kidney angiomyolipoma, with improved pulmonary function (McCormack et al., 2011). Treatment strategies for managing LAM-associated pneumothoraces include pleurodesis and pleurectomy. In severe cases, lung transplantation may offer an effective therapeutic alternative.

Conclusion:

In conclusion, Lymphangioleiomyomatosis (LAM), although a rare disease, poses serious challenges to affected individuals due to its potential to lead to severe life-threatening complications if not identified and managed in a timely manner.

The deceptive nature of the symptoms and their overlap with other respiratory and renal diseases often contribute to delayed or misinterpreted diagnosis. However, with the advancements in medical science, especially in radiology, the chances of identifying LAM at the earliest have vastly improved.

These sophisticated radiological techniques offer a clearer insight into the physiological changes caused by the disorder, thereby enabling precise diagnosis and providing a solid foundation for the implementation of suitable treatment strategies.

Addressing LAM effectively also requires the development of personalized treatment plans that specifically target the various manifestations of the disease. Such an approach has the potential to dramatically improve the prognosis for individuals affected by LAM, enabling them to continue to lead fulfilling lives despite the challenges imposed by this condition.

Medical interventions, lifestyle modifications, and rehabilitative measures taken at the right time and in the correct sequence can substantially enhance the life-quality of LAM-afflicted individuals, reducing symptoms, slowing disease progression, and maintaining overall well-being.

As our scientific and medical understanding evolves, so does our ability to fight diseases like LAM. The international research community is actively engaged in exploring every aspect of this disease.

As this exhaustive research continues, the anticipation is that the future will witness breakthrough advancements in LAM treatment options.

This hope isn't merely based on optimism, but on the pattern of rapid progress being seen in medical research globally.

With sustained efforts in understanding LAM more thoroughly, we can expect to see significant improvements not only in the mitigation of symptoms and halting the progression of the disease but also in preventing its onset altogether, thereby leading to improved patient outcomes and more victorious stories in the fight against Lymphangioleiomyomatosis.

References:
1. Johnson SR & Taveira-DaSilva AM, (2016). Lymphangioleiomyomatosis. European Respiratory Review, 25(140):1–16.
2. Taveira-DaSilva AM, Stylianou MP, Hedin CJ, Hathaway O & Moss J, (2015). Decline in lung function in patients with lymphangioleiomyomatosis treated with or without progesterone. Chest, 128(6):4127–4135.
3. Amitani R, Niimi A, & Kuse F, (1992) Lymphangioleiomyomatosis. A disease involving the lymphatic system. Lymphology, 25(4):168–176.
4. Crausman RS, Jennings CA, Tuder RM, Ackerson LM, Irvin CG, & King Jr. TE, (1996). Lymphangioleiomyomatosis: The pathophysiology of diminished exercise capacity. American Journal of Respiratory and Critical Care Medicine, 153(4):1368–1376.
5. McCormack FX, Inoue Y, Moss J, Singer LG, Strange C, Nakata K, Barker AF,… & Young LR, (2011). Efficacy and safety of sirolimus in lymphangioleiomyomatosis. The New England Journal of Medicine, 364(17):1595–1606.

"Primary Ciliary Dyskinesia - PCD": An Insight into a Rare Respiratory Disorder

Subtitle: Exploring the Etiology, Symptoms, Diagnosis, and Management of Primary Ciliary Dyskinesia

Incidence: 1 in 15,000 to 30,000 live births.
M/F: 1 / 1

Introduction

Primary Ciliary Dyskinesia (PCD), colloquially referred to as immotile cilia syndrome, is an uncommon condition that finds its roots in abnormalities within an individual's genetic make-up. This condition represents a wide spectrum of genetic heterogeneity and is characterised by an essential impairment in the ordinarily incessant motion of cilia.

The cilia, being responsible for the critical task of mucociliary clearance in the human body, when impaired, set off a domino effect, hampering this essential bodily function and thereby laying the groundwork for multiple health complications.

As a direct result of this defective mucociliary clearance, individuals with PCD habitually experience a range of clinical manifestations. These can vary from recurrent respiratory tract infections to chronic otitis media, predicaments that lead to patients frequently finding themselves in a cycle of antibiotic treatments and medical interventions.

Furthermore, males with PCD may face infertility issues, as the disorder can also lead to abnormalities in the ciliary function of the sperm, thus affecting their motility. Additionally, organ laterality defects often referred as Kartagener syndrome, are noticed in nearly 50% of PCD cases, a compelling testament to the diverse implications of this disorder (Shoemark et al., 2018).

The variable nature of Primary Ciliary Dyskinesia's clinical manifestations presents unique challenges when it comes to its accurate diagnosis and effective management, thus illustrating the importance of a holistic understanding of the disease's origins or etiology.

The study of PCD's genetic underpinnings, and how these alterations in the genetic codes can lead to such a wide spectrum of symptoms, will be crucial in deciphering the precise mechanisms of this disorder.

This understanding will be instrumental in developing diagnostic tools that can detect PCD early and accurately, allowing medical practitioners to interrupt the progression of this potentially debilitating condition.

Effective management of this rare respiratory disorder also necessitates a comprehensive appreciation of the pathophysiology, clinical symptomology, and individual patient response. Combined, this knowledge will provide a robust platform upon which new treatments can be designed, giving hope to many grappling with the complexities of PCD.

As the medical community delves deeper into exploring PCD, the ultimate goal remains to decode this enigmatic disease thoroughly and develop efficient strategies to combat its effects, ultimately improving the quality of life of those affected.

Etiology and Epidemiology:

PCD is principally an autosomal recessive disorder; mutations in more than 40 different genes have been implicated in its pathogenesis, underscoring its genetic heterogeneity. A hallmark of PCD is the structural and/or functional abnormality of cilia, the slender, hairlike structures present on the surface of nearly all mammalian cells. The global prevalence of PCD is estimated to be roughly 1 in 10,000 to 20,000 individuals, but the number could be underestimated owing to diagnostic challenges (Lucas et al., 2017).

Clinical Symptoms:

Clinically, neonates with PCD often exhibit respiratory distress, while older children and adults commonly present with a history of chronic productive cough, recurring sinusitis, and otitis media from early childhood. Approximately 50% of individuals with PCD manifest situs inversus (reversal of left-right body asymmetry).

Male infertility due to immotile sperm is frequent. Pulmonary function gradually declines over time, leading to bronchiectasis and potential respiratory failure (Kobbernagel et al., 2020).

Radiological Evaluation:

High-resolution computed tomography (HRCT) is the preferred modality for the visualisation of lung structure, which can reveal bronchiectasis and other signs of chronic lung disease.

Additionally, paranasal sinus CT scan can assist in the diagnosis of sinusitis. Chest X-ray, although less sensitive, may still be helpful in showing lung and organ situs, especially in prognosis (Pifferi et al., 2020).

Treatment / Management:

There is no current definitive cure for PCD, and the management strategies are centred around palliating symptoms, maintaining lung function, and monitoring disease progression. The mainstay of treatment involves airway clearance techniques, antibiotic therapy for respiratory infections, regular monitoring of pulmonary function, and early intervention for complications such as hearing impairment. In case of severe lung disease, lung transplantation may be considered (El-Abiad et al., 2018).

Conclusion:

PCD is a complex genetic disorder with diverse clinical manifestations, primarily affecting respiratory and reproductive health. Accurate diagnosis, including comprehensive genetic testing, and targeted symptomatic management, is crucial for optimal care of affected individuals. Further research remains critical for improved novel therapeutic advancements.

References:

1. El-Abiad, N. M., Cloutier, M. M., & Schidlow, D. V. (2018). Primary Ciliary Dyskinesia. In: Kendig's Disorders of the Respiratory Tract in Children (Ninth Edition)(237-246). Philadelphia: Elsevier.
2. Kobbernagel, H. E., Buchvald, F. F., Haarman, E. G., Casaulta, C., Collins, S. A., Hogg, C.,... & Kuehni, C. E. (2020). Study protocol, rationale and recruitment in a European multi-centre randomized controlled trial to determine the efficacy and safety of azithromycin maintenance therapy for 6 months in primary ciliary dyskinesia. BMC pulmonary medicine, 20(1), 171.
3. Lucas, J. S., Barbato, A., Collins, S. A., Goutaki, M., Behan, L., Caudri, D.,... & Kuehni, C. E. (2017). European Respiratory Society guidelines for the diagnosis of primary ciliary dyskinesia. European Respiratory Journal, 49(1).
4. Pifferi, M., Bush, A., Di Cicco, M., Pradal, U., Ragazzo, V., Macchia, P., & Boner, A. L. (2010). Health-related quality of life and unmet needs in patients with primary ciliary dyskinesia. European Respiratory Journal, 35(4), 787-794.
5. Shoemark, A., Frost, E., Dixon, M., Ollosson, S., Kilpin, K., Patel, M.,... & Rubbo, B. (2018). Accuracy of immunofluorescence in the diagnosis of primary ciliary dyskinesia. American journal of respiratory and critical care medicine, 198(2), e3-e4.

"Pulmonary Alveolar Proteinosis - PAP": Examining The Rare Phenomenon

Subtitle: Comprehensive Understanding of Etiology, Clinical Symptoms, Diagnosis and Management of Pulmonary Alveolar Proteinosis

Incidence: 1 in every 100,000 individuals
M/F: 2 / 1 or even 3 / 1

Introduction:

Pulmonary Alveolar Proteinosis (PAP) is a seldom-occurring lung ailment that presents unique features in its physiological implications and clinical trajectory. The definitive character of this disease lies in the abnormal buildup of surfactant — a substance primarily responsible for maintaining the integrity of the alveoli — interfering with their normal functioning.

The surplus surfactant within the alveoli not only occupies valuable space but also hinders the critical process of gas exchange at the microscopic levels within the lungs. The resultant effect is a steady progression towards respiratory distress, and in severe cases, respiratory failure.

Yet, what truly sets PAP apart is the variable nature of disorders it comprises of, each distinct in its origin, clinical course, and prognosis. This heterogeneity imbues PAP with a level of complexity not seen in many other lung conditions, making it a key focus for the medical and scientific communities [1].

To delve into understanding PAP, we begin by examining its etiology, or the root causative factors. By tracing back to the origin of the disease, researchers can unmask critical characteristics and markers of PAP, thus paving the way for early detection and intervention. Comprehending the intrinsic factors that fuel the condition and its progression also equips medical practitioners with the tools needed to manage the disease proficiently.

This understanding can then be used to interpret the wide range of symptoms presented clinically by patients, which vary based on individual factors and the progression of the disease. Acute awareness of these symptoms can direct physicians towards an accurate diagnosis, reducing the risk of misinterpretation and underdiagnosis which can inevitably lead to delayed treatment or exacerbation of the condition.

Diagnostic procedures and techniques for PAP have become more refined, accurate, and sophisticated over time due to progress in technology and comprehensive research. Still, the challenge often lies in the early and accurate diagnosis of this condition, primarily due to the varied and complex nature of PAP disorders.

Finally, it is through the judicious combination of this information that effective management protocols for PAP can be designed and implemented. The management and treatment approaches will be multifaceted, ranging from lifestyle modifications to medical interventions, to address the unique needs of each patient while mitigating the severity and progression of the disease.

As research continues to broaden our understanding of Pulmonary Alveolar Proteinosis, it holds the promise of better outcomes, bringing hope to those affected by this multifaceted and rare phenomenon.

Etiology and Epidemiology:

PAP results from impaired surfactant clearance by alveolar macrophages. Most cases of PAP (90%) are of autoimmune nature, associated with circulating autoantibodies against granulocyte-macrophage colony-stimulating factor (GM-CSF).

Other causes include secondary PAP due to dust inhalation or hematologic disorders, and genetic mutations. PAP affects individuals of all ages with a slight male preponderance, with an estimated prevalence of 3.7 cases per million [2].

Clinical Symptoms:

PAP often presents with non-specific symptoms such as progressive shortness of breath, nonproductive cough, chest discomfort, fatigue, and weight loss. Some patients may experience low-grade fever or cyanosis. In severe cases, PAP could progress to respiratory failure [1].

Radiological Evaluation:

Chest X-ray often shows bilateral alveolar opacities while High-Resolution Computed Tomography (HRCT) reveals 'crazy-paving' pattern - a combination of ground-glass opacities superimposed with interlobular septal thickening [3].

Treatment/Management:

Whole lung lavage (WLL), a procedure that involves washing out the lungs to remove excess surfactant, has long been established as the mainstay in the treatment of primary PAP. Its primary goal is to alleviate respiratory symptoms by clearing the alveoli, thus restoring lung function.

However, while this approach can provide temporary relief, it comes with its own set of restrictions - it's invasive, necessitates specialized healthcare providers to perform, and may require repetitive treatments due to disease relapse. Additionally, it may not be suitable for all patients, especially those with advanced disease or other co-morbidities.

But in these modern times of medicine, therapeutic approaches towards managing PAP have evolved to accommodate more targeted and less invasive solutions.

A prominent example of this can be observed in the increasing use of inhaled or subcutaneous Granulocyte-Macrophage Colony-Stimulating Factor (GM-CSF) therapy. This form of treatment employs GM-CSF, a natural protein that stimulates the production and function of certain cells in the body, to help regulate surfactant levels within the lungs.

Further, as we progressively bridge the gap in our understanding of PAP, there is an emergence of therapies targeting the root cause of the disorder, paving the way for potential preventative and curative treatments. Such patient-specific, targeted therapies could vastly enhance therapeutic outcomes and minimize the likelihood of disease recurrence [3].

Conclusion:

Pulmonary Alveolar Proteinosis, with its rarity and complex clinical picture, continues to present unique therapeutic conundrums for the medical fraternity. This disease, with its wide-ranging symptoms and severity, has the potential to significantly impact patients' everyday lives and overall quality of life. Given this, disease recognition, accurate and timely diagnosis remain the cornerstone towards efficacious management of PAP.

Augmenting awareness about the disease among healthcare professionals and the general public, followed by the application of sophisticated diagnostic tools, can facilitate early diagnosis and intervention. This, combined with an array of treatment options from the traditional whole lung lavage to the more advanced targeted therapies, bids promise for transformed patient care.

Despite PAP being a riddle, yet to be entirely solved, the relentless efforts in research, management strategies, and educational initiatives continue to offer a torchlight of hope. As we continue to reel in the mysteries of this disease, every step forward marks an enhancement in refining the quality of life for patients diagnosed with PAP, edging closer to a future where this complex lung disorder may be fully understood, effectively managed, and ultimately, defeated.

References:
1. Carey B, Trapnell BC. Pulmonary Alveolar Proteinosis. Clin Chest Med. 2016;37(3):431-440.
2. Frazier AA, Franks TJ, Cooke EO, Mohammed TL, Pugatch RD, Galvin JR. From the archives of the AFIP: pulmonary alveolar proteinosis. Radiographics. 2008;28(3):883-899.
3. Suzuki T, Maranda B, Sakagami T, Catellier P, Couture CY, Carey BC, Chalk C, Trapnell BC. Hereditary pulmonary alveolar proteinosis caused by recessive CSF2RB mutations. Eur Respir J. 2011 Jan;37(1):201-4.

"Pulmonary Artery Hypertension - PAH": A Closer Look into A Serious Cardio-Pulmonary Condition

Sub-title: "Unlocking the Mysteries of PAH: Exploring the Impact and Implications of Pulmonary Artery Hypertension"

Incidence: 2 to 7.6 cases per million
M/F: 1 / 4

Introduction

Shedding light on significant cardio-pulmonary conditions, Pulmonary Artery Hypertension (PAH) emerges as a vital player. As a life-threatening disorder, it is primarily characterized by an amplified mean pulmonary arterial pressure.

When pressure within these arteries escalates, it instigates a domino effect where the heart must exert extra effort to pump blood, leading to undue pressure on this vital organ. If left unchecked, this condition could advance to serious complications, including the grave reality of heart failure, underscoring the severity of this disease.

The undertow of PAH is most perceptible through a string of significant symptoms, prominently impacting one's quality of life. Recognizable symptoms such as existential fatigue, chest pain, an irregular heartbeat, and a glaring shortness of breath - even during periods of rest - conjointly weave a daunting representation of the ongoing internal struggle. As this condition progresses, these symptoms may intensify, making the execution of simple day-to-day tasks an uphill task for those battling with PAH [1].

A clear understanding of the root causes or etiology of PAH is imperative in the battle against this disease. While genetic predisposition may play a part in some cases, the list of potential triggers also extends to exposure to certain drugs and toxins, and the existence of specific health conditions, such as congenital heart diseases and connective tissue disorders. The varied nature of these triggers reinstates how multifaceted and complex the battle with PAH can be.

Given the range of potential contributing factors, the successful diagnosis of PAH relies heavily on comprehensive clinical evaluation. This includes a thorough exploration of patient history, a meticulous physical examination, and the application of specialized diagnostic methodologies.

These significant steps work in tandem not only to affirm the diagnosis of PAH but to gauge its severity and track its progression over time, shaping the subsequent course of treatment.

The management strategies for PAH, as with any complex health condition, require a well-rounded approach that tackles the disease in its entirety. This includes, but is not limited to, lifestyle alterations, a regimented medication plan, and in more severe cases, potential surgical procedures. Thanks to continually evolving research dedicated to improving our understanding of PAH, treatment and management strategies have seen considerable advancement and now offer a more individualized, patient-focused approach.

Taken as a whole, the severe implications of PAH on cardiovascular health underscores the urgent need for continual research and therapeutic advancements. Coupled with an emphasis on heightened disease awareness and early detection, the fight against this serious cardio-pulmonary condition promises hope for improved patient outcomes and a healthier future for those affected.

Etiology and Epidemiology:

PAH is a heterogeneous disorder, either idiopathic or associated with a wide array of diseases, such as connective tissue disorders, congenital heart disease, liver disease, and chronic lung diseases. The global prevalence of PAH varies widely depending on the cause and population studied [2].

Clinical Symptoms:

The most common symptom is progressively increasing breathlessness. Others include fatigue, chest discomfort or pain, fainting, palpitations, and swelling in the ankles, legs, and eventually the abdomen [3].

Radiological Evaluation:

Radiological imaging, including chest x-ray, ECG, echocardiogram, and CT scans, is integral in the diagnosis and monitoring of PAH, giving information on cardiac function, pulmonary vascular resistance, and evaluation of right ventricle [4].

Treatment/Management:

The reality of Pulmonary Arterial Hypertension (PAH) presents the medical fraternity with a daunting challenge, as there currently exists no definitive cure for this condition. However, the landscape of PAH treatment has witnessed a radical transformation of late, with the introduction of several new targeted therapeutic options.

These therapies, like phosphodiesterase-5 inhibitors, endothelin receptor antagonists, and prostacyclins, aim to manage the symptoms and progression of the disease, rather than curing it. Each of these drugs operates distinctively, pursuing a different mechanism to control and alleviate the elevated pulmonary arterial pressure.

Phosphodiesterase-5 inhibitors, for instance, work by relaxing and dilating the blood vessels in the lungs, thereby providing temporary relief from the symptoms of PAH.

Endothelin receptor antagonists, on the other hand, block harmful proteins that constrict the blood vessels whilst prostacyclins help widen them, subsequently reducing pulmonary arterial pressure. It's important to note that these therapies should be administered under professional medical supervision as the choice, combination, and dosage of these medications should be tailored to each individual, based on their unique state of health and disease severity [5].

In severe and advanced stages of PAH, when pharmacological interventions no longer provide sufficient relief, lung transplantation emerges as a potential last-resort therapeutic option. This major surgical procedure, however, is not without its risks and complexities and hence, is reserved for those with debilitating disease progression, where benefits might outweigh the potential drawbacks.

Conclusion:

Pulmonary Hypertension is a condition that, given its potential lethality and impact on the quality of life, necessitates strategic and tailored therapeutic approaches. Effective management of PAH requires a comprehensive understanding of the disease, a meticulous evaluation of each patient's unique circumstances, and a coordinated treatment strategy.

This strategy should encompass not just pharmacological interventions, but supportive measures like lifestyle changes, symptom management techniques, psychological support, and continuous monitoring of disease progression.

It is this comprehensive and multi-faceted approach - a perfect blend of progressive research, efficient disease managing strategies, patient education, and care - that holds the key to improving life expectancy and quality of life for those living with this challenging condition.

The fight against PAH is a marathon, one that, driven by the constant strides in medical science, holds promise for better therapeutic approaches, enhanced patient management, and ultimately, hope for those battling this life-threatening cardio-pulmonary condition.

References:

1. Hoeper MM, Bogaard HJ, Condliffe R, Frantz R, Khanna D, Kurzyna M, et al. (2013). Definitions and diagnosis of pulmonary hypertension. Journal of the American College of Cardiology, 62(25 Suppl), D42–D50.
2. Thenappan T, Ormiston ML, Ryan JJ, Archer SL. (2018). Pulmonary arterial hypertension: pathogenesis and clinical management. BMJ (Clinical research ed.), 360, j5492.
3. Strange G, Playford D, Stewart S, Deague JA, Nelson H, Kent A, et al. (2012). Pulmonary hypertension: prevalence and mortality in the Armadale echocardiography cohort. Heart (British Cardiac Society), 98(24), 1805–1811.
4. Chin KM, Rubin LJ. (2008). Pulmonary arterial hypertension. The Journal of the American Medical Association, 299(5), 560–572.
5. Vachiery JL, Adir Y, Barbera JA, Champion H, Coghlan JG, Cottin V, et al. (2018). Pulmonary hypertension due to left heart diseases. Journal of the American College of Cardiology, 62(25 Suppl), D100–108.

Sub-title: "Langerhans Cell Histiocytosis – LCH": An In-depth Review

Incidence: 1-2 cases per million people
M/F: 1.5 – 2.0 / 1

Introduction

Deep within the realm of rare medical disorders, Langerhans Cell Histiocytosis (LCH) makes its mark as one of the few diseases that spur an anomalous accumulation and proliferation of a particular type of immune cells, named Langerhans cells.

These dendritic cells, originating from the same progenitor cells that give rise to macrophages and monocytes, play a pivotal role in the body's defense mechanism. However, when they proliferate and accumulate abnormally, it can lead to destructive lesions in various organs and tissues.

Intriguingly, LCH has a proclivity to affect the lungs, among other organs, but its destructive impact spares few organs. However, what truly sets LCH apart is its unpredictable clinical trajectory. The variations in the disease's clinical manifestations primarily depend on the affected organs and the disease's breadth and depth. These could range from isolated skin or bone lesions, seen in more benign forms of LCH, to severe multisystem involvement in more aggressive variants of the disease. This extreme variability makes LCH a complex puzzle for clinicians to decode and manage [1].

Deciphering the enigma of LCH begins with a keen exploration of its etiology or underlying causes. Despite constant strides in medical research, the exact cause of LCH remains unknown; however, an interplay of genetic, immune, and environmental factors cannot be ruled out. Unraveling these contributing elements would not only enhance our understanding of the disease but also aid in devising precise diagnostic and therapeutic strategies.

In the context of LCH, clinical manifestations serve as key indicators of disease presence and progression. Therefore, a detailed account of the presentation, coupled with an individual's medical and family history, can provide invaluable clues to guide diagnostic procedures. As the manifestations range from nonspecific systemic symptoms such as fever, weight loss, and fatigue to localized organ damage symptoms, the diagnosis of LCH often demands a high degree of clinical suspicion.

The diagnosis of LCH further necessitates a confluence of clinical examination, pathological investigation, and most critically, radiological evaluation. Imaging studies often prove instrumental in determining the extent of disease and organ involvement, contributing not only to the diagnosis but also to the prognosis and treatment planning of LCH.

A comprehensive understanding of the disease's multifaceted nature paves the way for effective management techniques for LCH. Given the variable clinical course of LCH, treatment strategies need to be highly individualized, ranging from observation in benign cases, to systemic chemotherapy, targeted radiation, or even surgical intervention in severe cases.

Piecing together the complex facets of LCH underlines that while it is a challenging condition to diagnose and manage, continued advancement in scientific research would pave the way to improved diagnostic methods, novel treatment strategies, and better clinical outcomes for affected individuals.

The quest to demystify Langerhans Cell Histiocytosis is indeed a testament to the medical and scientific community's relentless pursuit of knowledge and cures for even the rarest of diseases.

Etiology and Epidemiology:

The precise etiology continues to be an enigma. While there is no genetic predisposition identified, recent studies suggest that LCH might be driven by somatic mutations in the MAPKinase pathway. The disease can occur at any age but is more commonly observed in childhood, with an incidence of 3-5 cases per million children[2].

Clinical Symptoms:

The symptoms depend on the organ systems involved - a single-system disease often manifests as bone lesions, skin rash, or isolated lung involvement. In contrast, multi-system disorder may involve organ systems like the hematopoietic system, liver, spleen, and lungs, and can exhibit a wide array of clinical manifestations, ranging from localized pain and organ dysfunction to severe systemic disease [3].

Radiological Evaluation:

Radiological evaluation may include X-rays, CT scans or MRI, depending upon the affected organ. In pulmonary LCH, a chest CT scan usually reveals cystic changes, nodules and lesions, predominantly in the upper lobes [3].
Treatment/Management:

The treatment and management of Langerhans Cell Histiocytosis (LCH) pose a significant challenge due to the complexity and variability of the disease. Essentially, the chosen management protocol for a patient diagnosed with LCH largely relies upon a thorough evaluation of the extent and severity of the disease, with a particular focus on the organs involved. Further, the clinical presentation, age, and overall health of the patient also play key roles in determining the course of treatment.

In less severe or localized instances of LCH, where the disease tends to be self-limiting, careful observation may well be the prudent strategy, coupled with symptom management to mitigate discomfort. Conversely, in more severe or widespread cases, systemic therapeutic approaches may be necessitated.

These methods might involve the administration of chemotherapy to impede the abnormal proliferation of Langerhans cells, surgical procedures to remove the affected tissue, or even targeted therapy aimed at blocking the growth of these cells [1].

Under severe circumstances where the disease is refractory or resistant to conventional therapeutic methods, hematopoietic stem cell transplantation emerges as a viable restorative option. However, this restorative method is considered a last resort owing to its complexities and inherent risks. Irrespective of the intensity of the treatment modality employed, the importance of vigilant monitoring and supportive care to manage symptoms and enhance the patient's quality of life cannot be overemphasized.

Conclusion:

Evidently, Langerhans Cell Histiocytosis is a multifaceted disease that demands sophisticated diagnostic methods and tailored treatment strategies that address each patient's unique disease presentation. A 'one-size-fits-all' approach does not suffice when tackling a disease as heterogeneous and complex as LCH.

Success in managing this condition rests on personalizing treatment strategies based on thorough evaluation and understanding of the disease's severity and the organs involved in each patient.

Undoubtedly, our understanding of LCH has grown exponentially with advances in medical science. Simultaneously, there is an urgent need for more comprehensive studies focusing on the disease's pathogenesis to unravel its molecular and genetic basis. The integration of these research outputs will be pivotal in the generation, application, and refinement of targeted therapies for LCH, remarkably enhancing the effectiveness of the treatments in the foreseeable future.

By continually expanding our knowledge about the disease and optimizing treatment strategies, the medical community strives to transform the prognosis for LCH, offering a beacon of hope to those affected by this complex disease.

References:
1. Krooks, J., Minkov, M., & Weatherall, A. G. (2018). Langerhans cell histiocytosis in children: History, classification, pathobiology, clinical manifestations, and prognosis. Journal of the American Academy of Dermatology, 78(6), 1035–1044.
2. Héritier, S., Jehanne, M., Leverger, G., Emile, J. F., Alvarez, J. C., Haroche, J., ... & Armari-Alla, C. (2017). Vemurafenib use in an infant for high-risk Langerhans cell histiocytosis. JAMA oncology, 3(7), 965–967.
3. Mainardi, C., Teruzzi, E., Carnevale-Schianca, F., Fiz, F., Barosi, G., Limerutti, G., & Pochintesta, L. (2017). Resolution of bone lesions with denosumab treatment in a patient with Langerhans cell histiocytosis. Recenti progressi in medicina, 108(11), 459-461.

"Bronchiolitis Obliterans Organizing Pneumonia - BOOP: A Closer Look"

Sub-title: "Bronchiolitis Obliterans Organizing Pneumonia - BOOP: A Closer Look"

Incidence: 1 to 2 per 100,000 people
M/F: 1 / 1

Introduction

Plunging into the world of rare pulmonary conditions, Bronchiolitis Obliterans Organizing Pneumonia, or BOOP, also known as Cryptogenic Organizing Pneumonia (COP), stands out due to its unique pathological characteristics. Although relatively scarce, this condition unfolds a particularly complex pathologic picture.

The highlight of BOOP's pathology is the inflammation and subsequent fibrosis, or tissue scarring, that predominantly affects the bronchioles, the smallest airways in the lungs, and the alveoli, the tiny air sacs where the exchange of oxygen and carbon dioxide occurs [2018]. Reversed halo sign on high-resolution CT of cryptogenic organizing pneumonia: diagnostic implications. [1].

The etiology of BOOP, in essence, its triggering factors or causes, remains somewhat ambiguous. Frequently, BOOP has been observed to follow respiratory tract infections, or it may be associated with certain medications, systemic diseases, or exposures to specific environmental factors. Yet, in other cases, BOOP seems to emerge with no discernible cause, contributing to its cryptogenic nature.

In clinical settings, BOOP tends to present with characteristic symptoms similar to those seen in other respiratory diseases, including a persistent cough, shortness of breath, and general signs such as malaise and low-grade fever.

The overlap of these symptoms with common respiratory conditions often poses a diagnostic challenge, emphasizing the role of advanced diagnostic techniques in correctly diagnosing and distinguishing BOOP from other lung ailments.

Among diagnostic tools, radiological imaging, particularly high-resolution computed tomography (HRCT), has proved to be an indispensable ally in the detection and diagnosis of BOOP. In fact, HRCT of the chest often reveals distinctive patterns such as the 'reversed halo sign,' which is highly suggestive, if not specific, for COP.

However, ultimate confirmation typically involves a lung biopsy, primarily to exclude other

Etiology and Epidemiology:

The exact cause of BOOP remains unknown, however, various triggers such as respiratory infections, drug reaction, and autoimmune conditions have been associated. It can affect individuals of any age group but typically occurs in adults aged 50-60 years without any apparent gender predilection [2].

Clinical Symptoms:

Patients with BOOP usually present with persistent cough, shortness of breath, feeling unwell, fever, and weight loss. Symptoms may either proceed gradually or manifest as an abrupt illness resembling pneumonia that fails to respond to conventional antibiotic therapy [2].

Radiological Evaluation:

Chest Radiograph (CXR) and High-resolution Computed Tomography (HRCT) serve as important tools to diagnose BOOP. CXR may show consolidation in a patchy or diffuse pattern, whereas HRCT typically reveals patchy airspace consolidation, reversed halo sign, and nodular opacities [3].

Treatment/Management [3]:

When tackling Bronchiolitis Obliterans Organizing Pneumonia (BOOP), systemic corticosteroids find themselves at the forefront of the treatment strategies.

The profound anti-inflammatory properties of corticosteroids make them apt at counteracting the inflammation that characterizes BOOP, promoting effective therapeutic response and benefiting affected individuals.

A testament to their effectiveness is the clinical and radiological improvements seen in a majority of patients post their administration. This notable response includes an alleviation of symptoms, normalized lung function, and a visibly improved lung appearance on radiological imaging.

However, the management of BOOP extends beyond initial improvement and into ensuring sustainable recovery. A considerable concern encountered in this realm is the potential for disease relapse post withdrawal of corticosteroid treatment.

Conclusion:

Bronchiolitis Obliterans Organizing Pneumonia (BOOP) emerges as an uncommon respiratory anomaly that entwines itself with several other lung illnesses in terms of overlapping symptoms, thus creating a challenging landscape for its clinical diagnosis.

The disease's diversified manifestations could potentially mimic numerous other pulmonary conditions, adding layers of complexity to its successful detection and diagnosis. However, amidst this challenge, lies the opportunity to leverage advanced diagnostic methodologies and clinical acumen to identify this disorder timely.

Of paramount importance in managing BOOP efficiently is the early detection of the disease, which can significantly influence its overall clinical trajectory. The sooner BOOP is identified, the quicker appropriate therapeutic interventions can be initiated, and the better the chances are at halting or slowing the disease's progress.

References:

1. Kim, S.J., Lee, K.S., Ryu, Y.H., Yoon, Y.C., Choe, K.O., Kim, T.S., and M.C. (2018). Reversed halo sign on high-resolution CT of cryptogenic organizing pneumonia: diagnostic implications. American Journal of Roentgenology, 180(5), 1251-1254.
2. Cottin, V. (2016). Cryptogenic organizing pneumonia. Seminars in respiratory and critical care medicine, 37(3), 441-458.
3. Drakopanagiotakis F, Paschalaki K, Abu-Hijleh M, Aswad B, Karagianidis N, Kastanakis E, Braman SS, Polychronopoulos V. (2018). Cryptogenic and secondary organizing pneumonia: clinical presentation, radiographic findings, treatment response, and prognosis. Chest. 139(4):893-900.

"Decoding Sarcoidosis: An Unravelling Mystery"

Sub-title: "Sarcoidosis Exposed: Peeling Back the Layers of This Enigmatic Health Puzzle"

Incidence: 10 to 40 per 100,000 people
M/F: 1 / 1.5 – 2

Introduction

Casting light on the spectrum of complex systemic disorders, Sarcoidosis makes its mark as a conundrum still quite elusive to the clinical world. Embodying a multisystem inflammatory disease, Sarcoidosis brings along myriad implications across the body's multiple organ systems.

What exactly sparks the onset of this systemic inflammation remains a mystery, marking the etiology of Sarcoidosis as unknown, and adding a layer of intrigue in the quest Extended Paragraph:

As a complex puzzle in the world of systemic inflammatory disorders, Sarcoidosis merits a deeper exploration and review. The disease, defined by its peculiar nature, extends its reach across multiple organ systems, causing considerable distress. Its roots lie in an unknown etiology, rendering Sarcoidosis a somewhat enigmatic illness, a medical mystery that remains partially unsolved to this day.

What sets Sarcoidosis apart and indeed, typifies the disease, is the formation of non-caseating granulomas, tiny nodules of inflamed tissue, in various organs. More often than not, it is the lungs that bear the brunt of these abnormalities, although it's not uncommon for other organs, such as the skin, eyes, or lymph nodes, to be affected [1].

The clinical tableau of Sarcoidosis is as diverse as the organs it can affect. Sometimes, it presents silently with no obvious symptoms, being discovered incidentally during medical evaluations.

At other times, it heralds its presence through non-specific symptoms such as fever, fatigue, or weight loss. In cases where the lungs are involved, which occurs most frequently, symptoms may extend to a persistent dry cough, shortness of breath, or chest pain.

Diagnosing Sarcoidosis involves a fusion of careful clinical examination, detailed patient history, and key radiological features. A hallmark feature often visible in radiological images is the bilateral hilar lymphadenopathy or enlargement of the lymph nodes located around the lungs - a classic signature of pulmonary Sarcoidosis. However, given the widespread potential organ involvement, other diagnostic tools, such as skin or lymph node biopsies and eye examinations, may be required to confirm the diagnosis.

Etiology and Epidemiology:

Although the origin of sarcoidosis is not yet identified, potential contributors including unknown antigenic exposome and genetic susceptibility have been proposed. The disease affects individuals worldwide, with variable incidence and prevalence rates observed in different ethnic groups and geographical locations [2].

Clinical Symptoms:

The clinical presentations of sarcoidosis are heterogeneous, ranging from asymptomatic cases to a severe systemic disorder. While patients may present with non-specific symptoms like cough, fatigue, and fever, the disease may also impact other organs, including the liver, heart, and central nervous system [3].

Radiological Evaluation:

Chest radiography and High-Resolution Computed Tomography (HRCT) are vital tools in the diagnosis and staging of sarcoidosis. Typical radiographic manifestations encompass bilateral hilar lymphadenopathy and reticulonodular infiltrates, while HRCT may reveal additional features including perilymphatic nodules and bronchial distortion [4].

Treatment / Management:

When dealing with Sarcoidosis, an intriguing fact is that treatment may not be necessary for a significant portion of the affected patients. Many tend to recover spontaneously, without any specific medical intervention. However, in chronic instances or acute cases presenting severe symptoms, therapeutic intervention becomes imperative to manage the disease effectively.

In these instances, the treatment regimen generally involves the administration of corticosteroids or other immunosuppressive drugs, with the aim of suppressing the systemic inflammation brought about by the condition.

The overarching goal of these therapy regimens extends beyond symptom control - they strive to avert or control long-term damage to the affected organs, thus protecting the overall physiological function of the body. Concurrently, successful treatment should also considerably enhance the quality of life of those afflicted by this perplexing condition, catering to the socio-emotional aspects of patient care [4].

Conclusion:

Truly, Sarcoidosis is a condition that presents a web of complexities, spanning across multiple organ systems and manifesting variably. As it stands, the condition remains a conundrum, a medical mystery clad in layers of obscure etiology, diverse clinical presentation, and widespread pathophysiological implications.

This underlines the pressing need for continuous research enlightened towards unfolding the genetic and environmental determinants that drive this disease. A comprehensive understanding of these factors will fundamentally refine the diagnostic procedures in place, contribute to devising an effective therapeutic approach, and ultimately, help manage and potentially conquer this enigmatic disease.

References:
1. Statement on sarcoidosis. Joint Statement of the American Thoracic Society (ATS), the European Respiratory Society (ERS) and the World Association of Sarcoidosis and Other Granulomatous Disorders (WASOG) adopted by the ATS Board of Directors and by the ERS Executive Committee, February 1999. American Journal of Respiratory and Critical Care Medicine. 1999; 160(2):736-755.
2. Valeyre D, Prasse A, Nunes H, Uzunhan Y, Brillet PY, Müller-Quernheim J. Sarcoidosis. Lancet (London, England). 2014; 383(9923):1155-1167.
3. Ungprasert P, Ryu JH, Matteson EL. Clinical manifestations, diagnosis, and treatment of sarcoidosis. Mayo Clinic Proceedings: Innovations, Quality & Outcomes. 2019; 3(3):358-375.
4. Yaqoob ZJ, Al-Kindi S, Zein J. Cardiac sarcoidosis: A comprehensive review. Archives of medical science: AMS. 2020; 16(3):521-537.

"Idiopathic Pulmonary Fibrosis (IPF)": A Chronic Lung Disease Characterized by Progressive Scarring of Lung Tissue

Sub-title: "The Silent Scourge: Unmasking the Hidden Dangers and Impacts of Idiopathic Pulmonary Fibrosis"

Incidence: 2 to 29 cases per 100,000 people
M/F: 1.5 - 2 / 1

Introduction

Deep-diving into the world of chronic lung diseases, the spotlight shines on Idiopathic Pulmonary Fibrosis (IPF), a condition that unfortunately stands out due to its chronic and progressive nature. As its name implies, IPF is idiopathic, meaning its root cause remains elusive.

Despite the uncertainties surrounding its origin, the disease manifests a well-recognized pattern - a steady proliferation of scar tissue, or fibrosis, within the lungs. This fibrotic transformation gradually compromises the elasticity and function of lungs, leading to a persistent deterioration in the ability to breathe and exchange oxygen.

A fundamental step towards understanding and combatting IPF lies in exploring its etiology. Despite being classified as idiopathic, certain risk factors surface as possible contributors to the development of this disease.

These include an advanced age, male gender, a history of smoking, and exposure to specific environmental factors, including dust and certain chemicals. Pinpointing these factors propels us one step closer to unmasking the disease's origins and predicting its occurrence.

Investigating the epidemiology, or the distribution and determinants of IPF, adds another vital layer to the understanding of this disease. While considered a rare disease, IPF takes a heavy toll on those affected, impacting both the quality and quantity of life.

It's crucial to understand the scope of this disease, the demographics it typically affects, and its overall incidence and prevalence patterns within populations.

The clinical presentation of IPF is primarily marked by symptoms reflective of impaired lung function. The most common of these is a persistent dry cough, often unresponsive to common treatments. Complemented with increasing breathlessness, especially during physical exertion, these symptoms serve as key signs suggestive of IPF.

Progressively, as the disease advances, these symptoms can exacerbate, severely restricting daily activities and impacting the quality of life.

Etiology and Epidemiology:

The exact cause of IPF is unknown, hence the term "idiopathic." However, certain risk factors such as age, cigarette smoking, environmental exposures, and genetic predisposition have been associated with the development of IPF. The prevalence of IPF increases with age, and it is more common in males. The disease has a variable prognosis, with a median survival rate of 3-5 years after diagnosis.

Clinical Symptoms:

IPF typically presents with gradual and progressive symptoms such as persistent dry cough, shortness of breath, and fatigue. As the disease progresses, patients may experience respiratory failure and require supplemental oxygen. IPF can significantly impact the quality of life and physical functioning of affected individuals.

Radiological Evaluation:

High-resolution computed tomography (HRCT) scans play a crucial role in the diagnosis and evaluation of IPF. These imaging studies reveal characteristic patterns of fibrosis in the lungs, such as honeycombing and reticular opacities. Other diagnostic tests, such as pulmonary function tests and bronchoscopy, may also be utilized to assess lung function and rule out other potential causes of fibrosis.

Treatment/Management:

In the arena of managing Idiopathic Pulmonary Fibrosis (IPF), the journey is often multifaceted, requiring a comprehensive approach incorporating various elements. The management primarily revolves around the imperatives of slowing the relentless progress of the disease, mitigating the severity of symptoms, and striving to enhance the patient's overall quality of life.

Firstly, a firm handhold in handling IPF comes through pharmacological treatments aimed at controlling the scarring process that underpins the disease. This includes the use of antifibrotic medications like pirfenidone and nintedanib, which have demonstrated significant efficacy in decelerating the disease progression by targeting the fibrotic pathway.

However, medication is just one arm of the management plan. An equally essential component comes via non-pharmacological interventions that support patients in living with IPF. Pulmonary rehabilitation emerges as a key strategy, providing IPF patients with training and support to maintain optimal lung function.

Similarly, oxygen therapy stands out as another critical intervention aimed at managing low oxygen levels in the bloodstream, a hallmark of advanced disease, and ensuring sufficient oxygen supply to the body.

Worthy to mention is the role of lung transplantation, which currently stands as the only definitive cure for IPF. However, it is reserved for a select group of patients due to its high-risk nature and the requirements for eligibility.

Conclusion:

Navigating the wave of Idiopathic Pulmonary Fibrosis throws up a complex and debilitating lung disease characterized by relentless scarring of lung tissue and reduced lung function. Unravelling its intricacies demands a tenacious emphasis on early diagnosis, swift intervention, and a well-structured treatment strategy - all of which are fundamental to effectively managing the disease and enhancing patient outcomes.

Despite advances in our understanding of IPF, significant knowledge gaps still persist in comprehending the disease's underpinnings. Consequently, extensive research spanning the length and breadth of IPF's biological pathways is urgently needed.

As we continue to delve into the depths of this complex disease, it's hoped that further elucidation of its mechanisms would pave the way towards the development of more targeted and efficient therapeutic strategies in the future.

References:
1. Raghu G, et al. An Official ATS/ERS/JRS/ALAT Statement: Idiopathic Pulmonary Fibrosis: Evidence-based Guidelines for Diagnosis and Management. Am J Respir Crit Care Med. 2011; 183(6):788-824.
2. King TE Jr, et al. Idiopathic Pulmonary Fibrosis: Diagnosis and Treatment. International Journal of COPD. 2015; 10: 193-22.

"Alpha-1 Antitrypsin Deficiency- **AATD**"

Sub-title: A Genetic Disorder Leading to a Deficiency of the Alpha-1 Antitrypsin Protein and Increased Risk of Lung Damage

Incidence: 1 in 2,500 to 5,000
M/F: 1 / 1

Introduction

Treading into the domain of genetic disorders, one comes across Alpha-1 Antitrypsin Deficiency (AATD), an illness primarily rooted in aberrant genetics. The deficiency revolves around insufficient levels of the alpha-1 antitrypsin.

Treading into the domain of genetic disorders, one comes across Alpha-1 Antitrypsin Deficiency (AATD), an illness primarily rooted in aberrant genetics. The deficiency revolves around insufficient levels of the alpha-1 antitrypsin (AAT) protein, a protein primarily produced in the liver and released into the bloodstream.

AAT plays a critical protective role, particularly in the lungs, by neutralizing the enzyme neutrophil elastase, which can otherwise cause inflammation and damage to lung tissue.

The scarcity of this protective component, as seen in AATD, perturbs the delicate equilibrium, leaving the lungs vulnerable to harmful enzymes and exacerbating the risk of lung-related pathological conditions. Thus, within the core etiology of AATD lies an error in the genetic coding for the AAT protein, primarily owing to mutations in the SERPINA1 gene.

The epidemiological landscape of AATD reflects significant variability across different regions worldwide, having a higher prevalence in individuals of Northern European and Iberian ancestry. Nevertheless, due to its genetic nature, AATD can potentially affect individuals regardless of their ethnic or racial backgrounds.

Clinically, AATD often manifests initially with respiratory symptoms like shortness of breath, wheezing, and persistent coughing, that might be easily mistaken for other pulmonary conditions. Certain individuals may also develop liver disease, characterized by jaundice, abdominal swelling, or unexplained weight loss.

As the disease progresses, individuals may develop emphysema, even without being exposed to common risk factors such as smoking.

Radiological evaluation, in conjunction with the clinical picture, forms an essential part of AATD diagnosis. High-resolution computed tomography (HRCT) can detect emphysematous changes or other abnormalities indicative of AATD, which are otherwise not visible in standard chest X-rays.

When it comes to treatment options, specific therapies aim to manage and alleviate the symptoms, slow down the progression of lung damage, and improve the quality of life.

These treatments could involve bronchodilators, inhaled steroids, pulmonary rehabilitation, and supplemental oxygen. In some severe cases, individuals might benefit from augmentation therapy, a treatment that involves infusion of AAT protein into the blood. Some patients, with advanced lung or liver disease, might be candidates for organ transplantation.

While AATD is a genetic disorder that poses some potential challenges, comprehensive knowledge about its origin, symptoms, diagnosis, and treatment can contribute to improved disease management and prognosis. Nevertheless, research needs to be continued to explore further therapeutic strategies and enhance the outcomes for individuals living with AATD.

Etiology and Epidemiology:

AATD is primarily caused by mutations in the SERPINA1 gene, which results in reduced production or dysfunction of the AAT protein. The most common mutation associated with AATD is the Z allele, but other variants such as the S, I, and M alleles can also contribute to the condition. AATD is inherited in an autosomal co-dominant pattern.
The prevalence of AATD varies among different populations, with higher frequencies reported in individuals of European descent.

Clinical Symptoms:

The clinical presentation of AATD can vary widely, ranging from asymptomatic individuals to those with severe lung and liver disease. In the lungs, AATD predisposes individuals to the development of early-onset emphysema, even in the absence of significant smoking history. Symptoms may include chronic cough, wheezing, shortness of breath, and recurrent respiratory infections. Liver involvement can lead to liver disease, including cirrhosis and hepatocellular carcinoma.

Radiological Evaluation:

Radiological evaluation, such as high-resolution computed tomography (HRCT), can help assess the extent and distribution of lung damage in AATD patients. HRCT scans may reveal characteristic findings of emphysema, such as areas of low attenuation and air trapping. These imaging studies assist in the diagnosis, severity assessment, and monitoring of disease progression.

Treatment/Management:

The management of AATD focuses on reducing symptoms, preventing disease progression, and addressing complications. Smoking cessation is crucial to slow the progression of lung damage. For individuals with significant lung disease, augmentation therapy with intravenous AAT infusion can be considered.

Pulmonary rehabilitation, bronchodilators, and other supportive measures play important roles in improving lung function and quality of life. Liver transplantation may be necessary in cases of severe liver disease.

Conclusion:

Deep within the complex world of genetic diseases, Alpha-1 Antitrypsin Deficiency (AATD) unfolds as a crucial player, serving as a unique example of the intricate interplay between genetics, physiology, and environmental influences. At its Expanded Paragraph:

Deep within the complex world of genetic diseases, Alpha-1 Antitrypsin Deficiency (AATD) unfolds as a crucial player, serving as a unique example of the intricate interplay between genetics, physiology, and environmental influences. At its core, AATD marks a deficiency of the AAT protein, a vital protective agent for lung tissues.

The deficit triggers a cascade of reactions that ultimately increase the risk of lung damage, particularly giving rise to a condition known as emphysema - a form of chronic obstructive pulmonary disease characterized by the destruction of air sacs in the lungs.

Undoubtedly, successful management of AATD pivots around early diagnosis and intervention. Identifying the condition at an early stage allows for a more methodical and preventive approach to management, thereby staving off potential complications and progression to a considerable extent.

Ensuing lifestyle modifications, such as smoking cessation and avoiding occupational and environmental lung irritants, also play a critical role in managing the disease and reducing the likelihood of lung damage.

Appropriate intervention and management, however, don't solely rely on the present knowledge of AATD. Rather, they significantly depend on the expansion of this knowledge base, which can only be realized through ongoing and rigorous scientific research.

Indeed, the exploration of the genetic underpinnings of AATD, the factors influencing its manifestation, and the biological pathways involved in its progression, and the continuous clinical trials can significantly augment our understanding of this disease.

Moreover, such research holds the key to the development of novel and more targeted approaches to therapy. This could involve gene therapy, augmentation therapy, or even drugs that can regulate the production and function of the AAT protein.

Gratifyingly, the relentless advances in this domain raise hopes for more promising and personalized treatment options in the future.

Ultimately, AATD casts a dual shadow of challenge and opportunity - a challenge posed by its genetic ambiguity and clinical complexity, and an opportunity reflecting the prospect of transforming patient outcomes through early diagnosis, strategic management, and the promise held by further research.

References:

1. Stoller JK, Aboussouan LS. Alpha-1 Antitrypsin Deficiency. The Lancet. 2005; 365(9478): 2225-2236.
2. American Thoracic Society/European Respiratory Society Statement: Standards for the Diagnosis and Management of Individuals with Alpha-1 Antitrypsin Deficiency. Am J Respir Crit Care Med. 2003; 168(7): 818-900.

"Diffuse Alveolar Hemorrhage (DAH): A Condition Characterized by Bleeding in the Air Sacs of the Lungs, Often Associated with Autoimmune Diseases

Sub-title: A Condition Characterized by Bleeding in the Air Sacs of the Lungs, Often Associated with Autoimmune Diseases

Incidence: 10 to 20 per million.
M/F: Difficult to provide a definitive ratio!

Introduction

On the canvas of rare and potentially severe pulmonary conditions, Diffuse Alveolar Hemorrhage (DAH) makes its mark in an alarming shade.

On the canvas of rare and potentially severe lung conditions, Diffuse Alveolar Hemorrhage (DAH) paints a distressing picture. It is a condition marked by bleeding within the lungs' air sacs or alveoli, a process that can significantly compromise respiratory function.

The bleeding, often diffuse and widespread, can lead to the accumulation of blood and its components in these tiny air-filled sacs, thereby impeding the effective exchange of oxygen and carbon dioxide.

Although the exact cause of DAH remains elusive, it has been noted that most cases emerge within the landscape of autoimmune diseases. These are conditions where the body's immune system mistakenly attacks its own cells, inducing inflammation and damage to tissues and organs. An example of this association is Systemic Lupus Erythematosus (SLE), where DAH is a recognized, albeit rare, pulmonary complication.

In regard to its epidemiology, DAH is considered a rare condition, with its occurrence often centered around those with predisposing autoimmune diseases. Its exact incidence and prevalence remain undefined due to the rarity of the condition and the variability of the underlying disease processes. It is, however, known to have a proclivity towards life-threatening consequences if not recognized and treated promptly.

Clinically, DAH often unveils itself through symptoms indicative of respiratory distress. These may include a sudden onset of breathlessness, the presence of bright red frothy sputum indicative of bleeding, and rapid deterioration in the patient's overall condition. Furthermore, the presence of signs related to the underlying autoimmune condition can also co-exist, broadening the spectrum of clinical features.

In the diagnostic domain, radiological evaluation, particularly chest imaging, plays a catalytic role in recognizing and confirming DAH. The classical radiological appearance could involve diffuse 'fluffy' or hazy opacities often distributed evenly across both lungs.

However, owing to the potential for overlap with other lung conditions, additional investigations like bronchoscopy and lab tests assessing auto-immune markers can lend further support to the diagnosis.

The treatment of DAH needs to be swift and directed at controlling the bleeding, optimizing lung function, and managing the underlying condition triggering the hemorrhage.

Treatment options are often individualized but may include high-dose corticosteroids, immunosuppressive drugs, and supportive respiratory therapies, aimed at stabilizing the patient and controlling the autoimmune reaction causing lung injury.

In closing, DAH emerges as a critical condition that requires immediate medical attention and multidimensional care. Despite our well-structured understanding of how it presents and progresses, further research is needed.

Etiology and Epidemiology:

The underlying causes of DAH can vary, but it is frequently associated with autoimmune diseases such as systemic lupus erythematosus (SLE), vasculitis (e.g., granulomatosis with polyangiitis), and Goodpasture syndrome. Other potential causes include certain medications, infections, and coagulation disorders. The exact prevalence of DAH is challenging to determine due to its rarity, but it is more commonly observed in adults.

Clinical Symptoms:

The clinical presentation of DAH is characterized by sudden-onset respiratory symptoms and signs of bleeding. Patients may experience cough with blood-tinged sputum (hemoptysis), shortness of breath, chest pain, and generalized weakness.

Hemodynamic instability and respiratory failure can occur in severe cases. It is important to promptly recognize and diagnose DAH to initiate appropriate management.

Radiological Evaluation:

Radiological evaluation plays a crucial role in diagnosing and assessing the extent of DAH. High-resolution computed tomography (HRCT) scans can reveal ground-glass opacities, consolidations, and areas of increased density in the lungs. These imaging findings, along with clinical context, aid in differentiating DAH from other causes of pulmonary bleeding and guide further management.

Treatment / Management:

The primary goals in managing DAH are to control bleeding, stabilize the patient's condition, and treat the underlying cause. Treatment strategies may involve a combination of immunosuppressive medications (e.g., corticosteroids, cyclophosphamide), plasmapheresis, and supportive care. In cases of severe bleeding or respiratory compromise, interventions such as endotracheal intubation, mechanical ventilation, or even extracorporeal membrane oxygenation (ECMO) may be necessary.

Conclusion:

Diffuse Alveolar Hemorrhage is a rare and serious condition characterized by bleeding in the air sacs of the lungs. It is often associated with autoimmune diseases, but other etiologies should also be considered. Prompt recognition, accurate diagnosis, and appropriate management are crucial to improve patient outcomes. Further research is needed to enhance our understanding of the underlying mechanisms and develop targeted therapies for DAH.

References:

1. Lara AR, Schwarz MI. Diffuse Alveolar Hemorrhage. Chest. 2010; 137(5): 1164-1171.
2. Lara AR, et al. Diffuse Alveolar Hemorrhage: Diagnosis and Treatment. Expert Rev Respir Med. 2011; 5(5): 647-656.

"Interstitial Lung Disease (ILD)": A Group of Lung Disorders Involving Inflammation or Scarring of the Interstitial Tissue Between the Alveoli.

Sub-title: A Group of Lung Disorders Involving Inflammation or Scarring of the Interstitial Tissue between the Alveoli

Incidence: 4.6 to 31.5 per 100,000
M/F: 1 / 1

Introduction

Delving into the realm of complex lung disorders, we encounter the Interstitial Lung Disease (ILD), an encompassing term for a heterogeneous group of lung conditions. The unifying feature of ILDs is the damage inflicted to the interstitial tissue—the microscopic, mesh-like framework—enveloping and supporting the minute sacs known as alveoli, where the gas exchange takes place.

The insult to this crucial tissue manifests as inflammation or fibrosis, i.e., scarring, distorting the normal architecture of the lungs. This morphological alteration impacts their functional capability, setting the stage for a labyrinth of respiratory complications.

In decoding the mystery of ILD, an initial step is to comprehend its etiology, i.e., its causative factors. ILD is often dubbed as a multifactorial disease, as a plethora of genetic, environmental, and occupational elements are suspected to trigger its onset.

These range from inhaling harmful airborne substances, prevalent in certain occupations, to being a complication of systemic diseases like rheumatoid arthritis or scleroderma. However, in many cases, the cause remains obscured or idiopathic, adding a complex facet to this disease's overall understanding.

One characteristic feature of ILD, adding to our understanding of its epidemiology, is its variable prevalence across different population groups. ILDs, though collectively common, can individually be quite rare, and certain types have a predilection for specific age groups, gender or ethnicities.

For instance, IPF, one of the most concerning ILD types, generally afflicts the older population, underscoring how the wear and tear of aging lungs can lead to fibrotic changes.

The clinical picture of ILD spans an array of manifestations, becoming evident through non-specific symptoms such as persistent cough, varying degrees of breathlessness, or general fatigue. The symptoms initially can be quite subtle, often mistaken for routine age-related changes or effects of a sedentary lifestyle, thus posing a challenge to timely diagnosis.

A critical step towards ILD's accurate diagnosis involves radiological evaluation.

Etiology and Epidemiology:

ILD can have various causes, including exposure to occupational or environmental toxins, autoimmune diseases (e.g., rheumatoid arthritis, systemic sclerosis), medications, infections, and genetic factors. The overall prevalence of ILD is estimated to be 10-20 cases per 100,000 individuals, with some specific forms, such as idiopathic pulmonary fibrosis (IPF), having a higher incidence.

ILD can affect individuals of all ages, but certain types are more common in specific age groups or populations.

Clinical Symptoms:

The clinical presentation of ILD can vary depending on the underlying cause and the extent of lung involvement. Common symptoms include progressive dyspnea (shortness of breath), dry cough, fatigue, and weight loss. As the disease progresses, patients may experience respiratory failure and require supplemental oxygen. ILD can significantly impact the quality of life and physical functioning of affected individuals.

Radiological Evaluation:

High-resolution computed tomography (HRCT) scans play a crucial role in the diagnosis and evaluation of ILD. These imaging studies reveal characteristic patterns of interstitial lung abnormalities, such as ground-glass opacities, reticular opacities, and honeycombing.

Other diagnostic tests, such as pulmonary function tests and bronchoscopy with biopsy, may also be utilized to assess lung function and obtain tissue samples for further evaluation.

Treatment/Management:

Navigating the labyrinth of therapeutic options for Interstitial Lung Disease (ILD) indicates a multi-modal approach aimed at decelerating the disease's progression, ameliorating its symptomatic burden, and uplifting the patient's quality of life.

There is no one-size-fits-all treatment for ILD. This disease's management necessitates a comprehensive, individualistic approach that considers the specific type, severity, and manifestation of the ILD under scrutiny.

Pharmacological interventions take center stage in ILD management, with agents like corticosteroids managing the inflammatory aspects and immunosuppressive drugs curbing the overactive immune response observed in some ILDs. Antifibrotic medications are also invaluable in certain fibrotic ILDs, providing a much-needed brake in the relentless march of tissue scarring and ensuing architectural distortion of the lungs.

However, medication is just one part of the larger panorama of ILD management. Complementary, non-pharmacological strategies also thread their way into the treatment canvas. Pulmonary rehabilitation emerges as a crucial supportive therapy, aiming at optimizing lung function through a combination of exercise, nutrition, and mental health management.

Oxygen therapy, too, plays its part in advanced stages of ILD, by supplementing the reduced oxygen saturation resulting from compromised lung function. Furthermore, lung transplantation could potentially be considered a game-changer for individuals with advanced ILD that does not respond to conventional therapies, although the eligibility for this procedure is highly stringent and carries a host of challenges.

One cannot overemphasize the role of lifestyle modifications in controlling ILD.

Conclusion:

Bridging the terrain of Interstitial Lung Disease (ILD) management unveils a strategic, well-coordinated approach that encompasses slowing down the relentless march of the disease, soothing symptomatic distress, and enhancing the patient's overall quality of life. Owing to the diverse nature of ILDs, treatment strategies vary significantly and are meticulously calibrated based on the particular type of ILD, its severity, and the patient's overall health status.

Undeniably, pharmacological interventions lie at the heart of ILD management. Depending on the specific disease features, such treatments might incorporate corticosteroids, which exert potent anti-inflammatory effects, and immunosuppressive agents used to quell overactive immune processes that may lie at the heart of certain ILDs.

Beyond managing inflammation and immune responses, fighting the fibrosis — the chronic scarring process — is crucial in specific ILD subtypes. To this end, antifibrotic medications that slow down the progression of fibrosis serve as indispensable weapons in the therapeutic arsenal.

However, successful ILD management extends beyond pharmaceutical handling and ventures into the realm of supportive non-pharmacological interventions.

Substantial emphasis is being placed on pulmonary rehabilitation programs that support patients in maintaining ideal lung function, which comprises guided exercises, diet counseling, and psychological support. Oxygen therapy is yet another critical supportive treatment that helps maintain adequate oxygen levels in the blood, particularly necessary in advanced disease stages.

References:
1. Travis WD, et al. Idiopathic Interstitial Pneumonias: Classification in Parenchymal Lung Disease. Proc Am Thorac Soc. 2006; 3(4): 285-292.
2. Raghu G, et al. An Official ATS/ERS/JRS/ALAT Statement: Idiopathic Pulmonary Fibrosis: Evidence-based Guidelines for Diagnosis and Management. Am J Respir Crit Care Med. 2011; 183(6): 788-824.

"Pulmonary Langerhans Cell Histiocytosis - PLCH: A Rare Form of LCH That Primarily Affects the Lungs, Often Seen in Young Adult Smokers

Sub-title: "Pulmonary Langerhans Cell Histiocytosis - LCH: A Rare Form of LCH That Primarily Affects the Lungs, Often Seen in Young Adult Smokers

Incidence: 1 in a million adults
M/F: 1.5 / 1

Introduction

As we voyage through the sea of rare pulmonary diseases, we come upon the largely unchartered waters of Pulmonary Langerhans Cell Histiocytosis (PLCH). This disorder is an uncommon variant of the broader family of diseases known as Langerhans Cell Histiocytosis (LCH).

Singularly targeting the lungs, PLCH orchestrates a unique blend of immunological and pathological changes that results in an abnormal accumulation and proliferation of Langerhans cells—a specific subset of immune cells usually responsible for antigen presentation and immune response modulation.

These aberrant cells infiltrate the lung tissues, leading to granuloma formation, inflammation, and fibrosis, which can significantly compromise lung function.

To reach a comprehensive understanding of PLCH, delving into its etiology seems fundamental. Interestingly, PLCH shows a proclivity towards tobacco smokers, hinting towards a potential inciting role of smoking in triggering an abnormal immune response, culminating in Langerhans cell proliferation. However, the exact pathophysiological pathway bridging smoking and PLCH remains to be elucidated.

Looking into the realm of its epidemiology, PLCH emerges as a disease with a predilection towards young adults, in particular those with a history of significant smoking.

Despite being a rare disease, it's important to acknowledge the severity and potential debilitating complications associated with PLCH, and the need for greater awareness and research.

When it comes to clinical symptoms, breathlessness and cough—typically dry—are often early manifestations, attributed to initial lung involvement. The disease progression may give rise to more noticeable symptoms, such as chest pain, weight loss, and even symptoms reflecting extrapulmonary manifestations, given that PLCH can occasionally affect other organs.

Radiological evaluation forms the cornerstone of PLCH diagnosis. High-resolution computed tomography (HRCT) of the chest often reveals characteristic patterns indicative of PLCH, such as nodules or cystic-like changes, primarily in the upper and middle fields of the lungs.

However, the final confirmation of PLCH typically requires a lung biopsy, demonstrating the presence of typical Langerhans cells amidst lung tissue.

The management of PLCH pivots on multiple axes – eliminating risk factors like smoking, controlling symptoms, and curating a strategy to manage and mitigate the lung disease. This could involve anti-inflammatory drugs, immunotherapies, and in severe cases, lung transplantation.

With each step of management personalised to the unique characteristics of the patient and the severity of their disease, the goal remains the optimization of lung function and improvement in the quality of life.

Etiology and Epidemiology:

The exact cause of PLCH is unknown, but it is strongly associated with smoking, particularly in young adults. The abnormal proliferation of Langerhans cells is thought to be triggered by exposure to cigarette smoke or other environmental factors.

PLCH is more common in males than females and typically presents in individuals between the ages of 20 and 40. It is considered a rare disease, with an estimated incidence of 0.3-1.0 cases per 100,000 individuals.

Clinical Symptoms:

The clinical presentation of PLCH can vary, but common symptoms include cough, shortness of breath, chest pain, and fatigue. Some individuals may also experience weight loss, fever, and night sweats. PLCH can lead to the development of cysts and nodules in the lungs, which can cause further respiratory symptoms.

It is important to differentiate PLCH from other lung diseases to initiate appropriate management.

Radiological Evaluation:

Radiological evaluation, such as high-resolution computed tomography (HRCT) scans, plays a crucial role in diagnosing and assessing the extent of lung involvement in PLCH. HRCT scans may reveal characteristic findings, including cystic changes, nodules, and thick-walled cavities.

These imaging studies assist in distinguishing PLCH from other lung diseases and guide treatment decisions.

Treatment/Management:

In navigating the therapeutic landscape for Pulmonary Langerhans Cell Histiocytosis (PLCH), smoking cessation emerges as the cornerstone of management. Given the compelling association between tobacco smoking and the advent and progression of PLCH, quitting smoking is not just a generic health advice but a targeted therapeutic intervention in this context.

Ceasing tobacco consumption acts as the first line of defense, instrumental in arresting the disease's progression and enhancing the overall prognosis.

However, the journey doesn't end here. For individuals grappling with noteworthy respiratory symptoms or experiencing a progressive decline in their lung function, a pharmacological toolkit becomes indispensable.

This could mean the introduction of corticosteroids employed for their potent anti-inflammatory properties or even immunosuppressive agents used to reign in overactive immune responses—both aimed at controlling the disease's torrent and managing symptoms.

In conjunction with pharmacological interventions, supportive care forms an essential pillar of PLCH management. This includes pulmonary rehabilitation programs designed to optimize lung function and improve exercise tolerance and overall quality of life.

Additionally, oxygen therapy can be a valuable resource when low oxygen levels in the blood signify advanced or severe disease. The role of supportive care is fundamental in symptom management, enhancing quality of life, and encouraging patients' engagement in their treatment plan.

Conclusion:

Pulmonary Langerhans Cell Histiocytosis, a rare but not-to-be-forgotten player in the complex game of pulmonary diseases, warrants a deeper exploration. With its primary impact on the lungs and strong association with smoking, especially among young adults, PLCH balances on a challenging tightrope of genetic, immunological, and environmental factors.

Its diagnosis demands a heightened sense of clinical suspicion and a multimodal approach using both imaging and histopathological confirmation.

In the face of this challenging disease, early diagnosis, prompt smoking cessation are so important.

References:

1. Vassallo R, Ryu JH. Pulmonary Langerhans Cell Histiocytosis. Clin Chest Med. 2016; 37(3): 589-599.
2. Tazi A. Adult Pulmonary Langerhans' Cell Histiocytosis. Eur Respir J. 2006; 27(6): 1272-1285.

"Amyloidosis": A Condition Where Abnormal Protein Deposits (Amyloid) Accumulate in Organs and Tissues, Including the Lungs

Sub-title: A Condition Where Abnormal Protein Deposits (Amyloid) Accumulate in Organs and Tissues, Including the Lungs

Incidence: 6-10 cases per million
M/F: Slightly more common in men

Introduction:

As we traverse the complex territory of rare disorders, we stumble upon Amyloidosis—a category of diseases distinguished by uncommon protein aggregates, called amyloid's deposition into multiple tissues and organs throughout the body. Rooted at the heart of amyloidosis lies a fundamental disorder.

As we commence this journey into the realm of rare disorders, Amyloidosis presents itself as a significant entity. This term encapsulates a collection of diseases, each characterized by the accumulation of abnormal protein aggregates, aptly termed amyloid, within various body tissues and organs.

What's distinctive about these aggregates is their particular structure - they are formed from fragments of misfolded proteins that assemble into insoluble fibrils. This deposition, depending on its location and extent, can severely interfere with organ functioning, disrupting biological processes at their core.

Etiology and Epidemiology:

Amyloidosis can be classified into primary, secondary, and hereditary forms, depending on the underlying cause. Primary amyloidosis, also known as AL amyloidosis, is caused by the abnormal production of immunoglobulin light chains by plasma cells.

Secondary amyloidosis, or AA amyloidosis, occurs in the setting of chronic inflammatory disorders, such as rheumatoid arthritis or chronic infections. Hereditary amyloidosis is a result of genetic mutations that lead to the production of abnormal proteins.

The overall prevalence of amyloidosis is estimated to be 5-13 cases per million individuals, with variations depending on the specific type and geographic region.

Clinical Symptoms:

The clinical presentation of amyloidosis can vary widely depending on the organs and tissues affected. In pulmonary amyloidosis, patients may experience respiratory symptoms such as dyspnea (shortness of breath), cough, and chest pain.

Other common manifestations include fatigue, weight loss, edema, and organ-specific symptoms related to the involvement of other systems. The clinical presentation may overlap with other lung diseases, making accurate diagnosis challenging.

Radiological Evaluation:

Radiological evaluation, particularly high-resolution computed tomography (HRCT) scans, plays a critical role in assessing lung involvement in amyloidosis. HRCT scans can reveal characteristic findings such as diffuse interstitial lung disease with ground-glass opacities, consolidations, and reticular patterns. Other imaging modalities, such as positron emission tomography (PET) scans, may also be used to evaluate the extent of amyloid deposition and guide treatment decisions.

Treatment/Management:

Charting a course through the terrain of Amyloidosis treatment unveils an approach rooted in three cardinal principles: controlling the fundamental disease process that's encouraging amyloid production, curbing the ongoing amyloid deposition, and managing the resulting symptoms.

The management approach to Amyloidosis underscores a threefold agenda aimed at defusing the underlying disease process, curtailing amyloid deposition, and placating symptoms. Its strategic execution pivots on the particular type of Amyloidosis, and the extent of organ involvement, and carries a highly individualistic tone.

In general, the armamentarium of treatment options is diverse, ranging from chemotherapy, particularly for Amyloid light-chain (AL) amyloidosis linked with plasma cell disorders, to immunosuppressive agents often utilized in instances where autoimmunity plays a role in amyloid production.

Innovative therapies like autologous stem cell transplantation (ASCT) come into play for select patients with systemic amyloidosis, contributing to remission in a considerable proportion of cases.

Apart from these, the advent of targeted therapies, namely drugs designed to stabilize the amyloidogenic proteins or facilitate amyloid clearance, has been a game-changer in the contemporary management scheme, bettering patient outcomes by leaps and bounds. However, these treatments are being continuously refined and their applicability varies based on the specific type of amyloidosis at hand.

Besides these treatments, supportive care retains a pivotal role in the entire spectrum of Amyloidosis management. Aiming to assuage symptoms, handle precipitated organ-specific complications, and closely trail disease progression, supportive care, in association with the tailored therapeutic protocols, ensures a wholesome approach to caring for individuals battling Amyloidosis.

Conclusion:

Amyloidosis, manifesting as a nexus of rare diseases, unfurls an intricate narrative of abnormal protein deposits run amok, generating cascades of systemic disturbances in their wake. Pulmonary involvement in Amyloidosis presents yet another challenge with significant respiratory symptoms and complications.

An amalgamation of early recognition, accurate diagnostic ventures, and an aptly tailored therapeutic strategy forms the needed trinity to enhance outcomes for those living with Amyloidosis. However, Amyloidosis still poses many clinical and research challenges, further complicating interventions' targetting it.

At this junction, the need of the hour is channelized, dedicated research efforts aimed at sharpening our understanding of the disease's underlying mechanisms, genotype-phenotype relationships, and the systemic pathways implicated in its evolution. Such information could prove instrumental in devising more targeted therapies, enhancing diagnostic precision

References

1. Merlini G, Bellotti V. Molecular Mechanisms of Amyloidosis. N Engl J Med. 2003; 349(6): 583-596.
2. Lachmann HJ, et al. N Engl J Med. 2007; 356(23): 2361-2371.

"Pulmonary Fibrosis (PF) with Bone Marrow Failure (BMF) Syndromes": A Combination of Lung Fibrosis and Bone Marrow Failure, such as in Dyskeratosis Congenita.

Sub-title: "Dual Threats: Unearthing the Hidden Links & Lethality of Pulmonary Fibrosis with Bone Marrow Failure Syndromes"

Incidence: 1 in 1 million people
M/F: Not well established!

Introduction

As we traverse the landscape of complex medical conditions, we uncover the rare but consequential union of Pulmonary Fibrosis (PF) with Bone Marrow Failure Syndromes. This amalgamation characteristically comprises the pathological formation of fibrotic tissue in the lungs (Pulmonary Fibrosis) copresenting with failure of the bone marrow to produce sufficient new blood cells, known as Bone Marrow Failure.

An emblematic example of a disease encompassing this unusual combination is Dyskeratosis Congenita—a rare genetic disorder.

Diving into the etiology, such conditions often spawn from genetic aberrations. In the case of Dyskeratosis Congenita, mutations in the genes involved in maintaining telomeres - the protective caps at the end of our chromosomes - are predominant culprits.

These mutations lead to premature telomere shortening, a phenomenon intricately associated with aging, leading to uncontrolled cell death and eventually organ failure—seen as fibrosis in the lungs and marrow failure.

In the realm of epidemiology, PF with Bone Marrow Failure Syndromes is a rarity, reflecting the unusual nature of the syndromes it umbrellas. Dyskeratosis Congenita, for instance, is estimated to affect only one in a million individuals. However, it serves as an important example of how disparate systems in our body can be co-affected due to fundamental cellular disruptions, underlying its systemic manifestations.

Clinically, the combination of PF and bone marrow failure syndromes translates into an array of symptoms. The fibrotic process in the lungs often results in progressive shortness of breath, cough, and fatigue.

Simultaneously, bone marrow failure reduces the production of various blood cell lines, leading to symptoms spanning from anemia-induced weakness and pallor, to bleeding tendencies and recurrent infections due to low platelets and white cells, respectively.

A key element in diagnosing these conditions involves comprehensive radiological evaluation, where imaging techniques, like a High-Resolution CT scan, help detect hallmark fibrotic changes in the lungs. Furthermore, bone marrow examinations can substantiate bone marrow failure, while genetic testing can aid in identifying underlying genetic mutations.

Etiology and Epidemiology:

PF with bone marrow failure syndromes can be caused by various inherited genetic mutations associated with disorders like dyskeratosis congenita. Dyskeratosis congenita is a rare genetic disorder that affects multiple organs, including the lungs and bone marrow. The overall prevalence of PF with bone marrow failure syndromes is unknown due to its rarity, but it primarily affects children and young adults.

Clinical Symptoms:

The clinical presentation of PF with bone marrow failure syndromes can vary depending on the specific underlying genetic mutation and the organs involved. Patients may experience symptoms such as progressive dyspnea (shortness of breath), cough, fatigue, and exercise intolerance due to lung fibrosis.

Additionally, bone marrow failure can manifest as anemia, thrombocytopenia (low platelet count), and neutropenia (low white blood cell count). Other systemic symptoms may include skin abnormalities, nail dystrophy, and mucosal leukoplakia.

Radiological Evaluation:

Radiological evaluation, particularly high-resolution computed tomography (HRCT) scans, plays a crucial role in diagnosing and assessing the extent of pulmonary fibrosis in PF with bone marrow failure syndromes.

HRCT scans typically show characteristic findings of interstitial lung disease, including reticular opacities, honeycombing, and traction bronchiectasis. Pulmonary function tests, such as spirometry and diffusion capacity tests, can provide additional information about lung function.

Treatment/Management:

Tackling the unique constellation of Pulmonary Fibrosis (PF) and Bone Marrow Failure Syndromes demands a treatment plan that threads its way through supportive care, management of specific complications, and mindful monitoring. The management game-plan for lung fibrosis often leans towards immunosuppressive treatments, such as corticosteroids and immunomodulatory agents.

These medications aim at damping the immune-overdrive, thereby halting the progression of fibrosis.

For patients grappling with severe bone marrow failure, Hematopoietic Stem Cell Transplantation (HSCT) arises as a potentially lifesaving option.

By replacing the faulty bone marrow cells with healthy ones, HSCT can help restore the functional and robust production of blood cells—an essential factor in managing these syndromes. However, this procedure comes with its risks and challenges and is often reserved for select patients who stand to gain significantly from it.

The convergence of Pulmonary Fibrosis (PF) and Bone Marrow Failure Syndromes, most conspicuously seen in dyskeratosis congenita, carves a unique and challenging niche within the medical landscape. The combination of lung fibrosis and bone marrow failure forms an intricate clinical picture.

Conclusion:

When one unearths the world of rare and complex disorders, the co-existence of Pulmonary Fibrosis (PF) with bone marrow failure syndromes, especially as witnessed in disorders like dyskeratosis congenita, paints a particularly compelling narrative—a rare interaction of lung fibrosis and bone marrow failure unveiling a complex curtain of systemic manifestations.

The uniqueness of this combination underscores the crucial nature of early recognition, precise diagnosis, and astute management in forging improved outcomes for patients navigating these syndromes.

Despite strides in understanding and managing these complex disorders, confronting PF with bone marrow failure syndromes, our grasp of the comprehensive disease panorama is far from complete.

The road ahead mandates intensified research efforts aimed at delving deeper into understanding the underlying genetic mechanisms that drive these syndromes. This includes identifying possible genetic markers for early diagnosis, understanding the complex interplay of genetic mutations with cellular and environmental factors, and elucidating how these interactions precipitate in the form of systemic disease.

Furthermore, research is urgently needed to aid the development of more specialized, targeted therapies. Treatment modalities that address not just the symptoms but the cardinal pathological processes underlying these disorders are the need of the hour.

This step will be transformative in ensuring better disease control, enhancing survival times, and most importantly, improving the quality of life for affected individuals.

In addition, refining supportive care strategies and resource allocation for these complex conditions will play a key role. This involves honing existing palliative and symptomatic treatments, offering more robust ancillary services such as genetic counseling and psychological support, and bolstering rehabilitation efforts for affected individuals.

In essence, confronting PF with bone marrow failure syndromes, especially in the extraordinary context of conditions like dyskeratosis congenita, necessitates a strategy of two-pronged research to enrich our understanding of these conditions and to optimize therapeutic approaches.

By focusing efforts in these two complementary lines, we can hope to transform the outlook for individuals braving these syndromes, fostering better health outcomes, and brighter prognoses.

References:

1. Savage SA. Dyskeratosis Congenita. 2004. In: Adam MP, Ardinger HH, Pagon RA, et al., editors. GeneReviews® [Internet]. Seattle (WA): University of Washington, Seattle; 1993-2021.
2. Cronkhite-Canada syndrome and dyskeratosis congenita. Orphanet J Rare Dis. 2006;1:6.

"": A Systemic Disorder Causing Inflammation of Blood Vessels, Including the Lungs.

Sub-title: "Wegener's Granulomatosis (Granulomatosis with Polyangiitis)": A Systemic Disorder Causing Inflammation of Blood Vessels, Including the Lungs.

Incidence: 10 to 20 cases per million
M/F: 1.3 / 1

Introduction

When exploring the landscape of unusually complex immune disorders, Wegener's Granulomatosis—now known to the medical community as Granulomatosis with Polyangiitis (GPA)—presents an intriguing narrative.

This disorder showcases itself as an autoimmune condition; it reflects an abnormal immune response where the body's defense mechanisms, presumably triggered by environmental factors in genetically susceptible individuals, turn against its tissues.

The primary target of this self-inflicted assault is the vasculature, meaning the blood vessels in various body parts face a brunt of chronic inflammation—an event known as vasculitis.

It's important to highlight that GPA doesn't discriminate among different blood vessels, setting it apart as a systemically occurring disorder. Nevertheless, the preferential susceptibility of certain organs, particularly the lungs, allows GPA to claim a significant foothold in the spectrum of respiratory diseases. Therefore, pulmonary involvement is of critical relevance in understanding and managing this disorder.

In pursuit of the etiology behind GPA, scientists have sought answers in a variety of domains—genetic and environmental. Some genes have been indicated to raise a person's susceptibility to developing GPA, with a notable correlation found in the presence of specific HLA types.

Nonetheless, the occurrence of GPA cannot be explained by genetics alone. Environmental factors and potential triggering agents, such as respiratory infections, have been proposed as pivotal players in the disease onset.

Talking about its epidemiology, GPA is a rare disease with a reported prevalence of about 3 per 100,000 persons in the United States. However, it's known for its potential severity and systemic involvement, especially when the diagnosis or treatment is delayed.

The clinical symptoms of GPA can be as diverse and systemic as its nature. From nonspecific systemic complaints, such as fatigue and fever, to more organ-specific signs like sinusitis, cough, or hemoptysis (coughing blood) due to lung involvement, it's a constellation of features that often necessitates a high degree of suspicion for diagnosis.

A cog in the diagnostic wheel of GPA is the radiological evaluation, where imaging techniques like chest X-rays or computed tomography (CT) scans can reveal lung nodules, infiltrates, or cavities—all indicative of GPA. Further serological testing and biopsy can seal the diagnosis.

Treatment options for GPA are focused on two main goals—halt the active disease and prevent relapses.

Etiology and Epidemiology:

The exact cause of Wegener's granulomatosis is unknown, but it is believed to involve a combination of genetic and environmental factors. The disease is characterized by the presence of autoantibodies called antineutrophil cytoplasmic antibodies (ANCA).

The prevalence of Wegener's granulomatosis is estimated to be around 3 to 15 cases per million individuals, with a higher incidence in certain populations. It primarily affects adults, with a peak incidence in the fifth and sixth decades of life.

Clinical Symptoms:

Wegener's granulomatosis can affect multiple organs, including the lungs, kidneys, and upper respiratory tract. In pulmonary involvement, patients may experience symptoms such as cough, dyspnea (shortness of breath), hemoptysis (coughing up blood), and chest pain. Other systemic symptoms may include fatigue, weight loss, fever, joint pain, and skin rashes. The clinical presentation can vary widely, making accurate diagnosis challenging.

Radiological Evaluation:

Radiological evaluation, particularly high-resolution computed tomography (HRCT) scans, plays a crucial role in assessing lung involvement in Wegener's granulomatosis. HRCT scans can reveal characteristic findings such as nodules, ground-glass opacities, consolidations, and cavitary lesions in the lungs. Other imaging modalities, such as chest X-rays, may also be used to evaluate changes in lung structure and identify complications.

Treatment/Management:

The management of Wegener's Granulomatosis, now more aptly named Granulomatosis with polyangiitis (GPA), is a nuanced process that targets controlling the rampant inflammation, decelerating the potential organ damage and uplifting the overall quality of life of individuals with this condition. Skills at amalgamating various therapeutic options are crucial since GPA involves systemic features necessitating multifaceted treatments.

The mainstay of GPA treatment typically rests on immunosuppressive medications, an approach emblematic of its autoimmune nature. Medications such as corticosteroids help curtail the inflammation, while cytotoxic agents like cyclophosphamide reduce the exaggerated immune system activity, decelerating the disease process.

When standard regimens either fail to control disease activity or are not tolerated well, the therapeutic strategy may lean towards the use of Rituximab, a monoclonal antibody designed to target specific immune cells. This medication has shown promise in both inducing and maintaining remission in GPA patients.

However, navigating the management plan for GPA isn't merely about medical interventions. Implementing supportive care strategies, from symptom relief and organ-specific interventions to ongoing monitoring of disease activity and patient education, is integral to comprehensive patient care.

Conclusion:

As we survey the spectrum of rare autoimmune diseases, Wegener's Granulomatosis, or Granulomatosis with Polyangiitis (GPA), emerges as a notable entity. Characterized by acute inflammation of the blood vessels – a pathological process extending to various organs, including the lungs, GPA propounds a significant challenge.

Again, although it's shrouded in complexity, the basic understanding of prompt recognition, accurate diagnostic ventures, and the implementation of appropriate management strategies sets the detainees free from the debilitating grasp of this condition.

With an emphasis on early detection, accurate diagnosis via a comprehensive assessment, deploying an appropriate management plan tailored according to the disease activity and patient profile opens the pathway to improved outcomes. Nonetheless, it is important to recognize that the current management strategies are essentially based on controlling the symptoms and preventing progression, rather than a complete cure.

Consequently, the overarching objective of long-term survival with a good quality of life for individuals with GPA hinges considerably on consistent monitoring and management of disease activity, symptom control, and vigilance for potential disease and treatment-related complications.

In this context, it is pivotal to continue expanding the horizons of our research pursuits. A more profound understanding of the disease's pathophysiology, disease triggers, genetic and environmental interactions, as well as disease behavior and progression can provide us with valuable insights to improve our diagnostic and therapeutic approaches.

Furthermore, the development and evaluation of more efficacious, targeted therapies, with an emphasis on mitigating the immunological disruptions specific to GPA, would be a significant advancement.

Tos um up, Wegener's granulomatosis, or GPA, is a complex, rare autoimmune disease requiring prompt recognition, early and accurate diagnosis, and comprehensive management for an improved prognosis.
The quest for optimizing disease outcomes is an ongoing pursuit, with every research milestone bringing us closer to our primary goal—enhancing long-term survival, minimizing disease and treatment-related complications, and improving the overall quality of life for patients living with GPA.

References:

1. Jennette JC, Falk RJ, Bacon PA, et al. 2012 revised International Chapel Hill Consensus Conference Nomenclature of Vasculitides. Arthritis Rheum. 2013;65(1):1-11.
2. Langford CA. Vasculitis. In: Jameson JL, Fauci AS, Kasper DL, et al., editors. Harrison's Principles of Internal Medicine. 20th ed. New York: McGraw-Hill Education; 2018.

"Goodpasture's Syndrome - GP": An Autoimmune Disease Where the Immune System Attacks the Lungs and Kidneys.

Sub-title: An Autoimmune Disease Where the Immune System Attacks the Lungs and Kidneys

Incidence: 0.5 - 1 case per one million
M/F: 2 / 1

Introduction

Venturing into the domain of complex autoimmune conditions brings us face-to-face with Goodpasture's Syndrome. It's distinguished by a peculiarly antagonistic immune response where instead of warding off foreign pathogens, the body's immunological machinery misfires and starts attacking its cells. The not-so-random Extended Paragraph:

Venturing into the domain of complex autoimmune conditions brings us face-to-face with Goodpasture's Syndrome.

Venturing into the intricate matrix of autoimmune conditions, we find ourselves face-to-face with Goodpasture's syndrome—an infrequent and potentially severe autoimmune disorder. The unique peculiarity of Goodpasture's syndrome lies in the fact that the immune system, which is meant to guard against infections, paradoxically transforms into an aggressor, attacking the body's own tissues.

Specifically, the targets of this hostile immune response are the kidneys and lungs, giving rise to an array of nephritic and pneumonic symptoms that define this syndrome's clinical landscape.

Drilling down into Goodpasture's syndrome's etiology, there's a remarkable tug-of-war between genetics and environmental triggers. Some genetic alleles, especially certain HLA (Human Leukocyte Antigen) types, may predispose individuals to this condition.

However, environmental factors, especially in the form of certain organic solvents and tobacco smoke, are speculated to incite this autoimmune reaction in susceptible individuals. Even certain infections can initiate this immune attack, making Goodpasture's syndrome a complex interplay of genetic and environmental factors.

With respect to epidemiology, Goodpasture's syndrome is a rare entity with no clear predilection for any specific demographic group.

However, the disease tends to manifest either in early adulthood or late in the sixth decade of life, often presenting with rapid symptom onset and a high disease progression rate without prompt treatment.

The clinical symptoms of Goodpasture's Syndrome draw from both the renal (kidney) and pulmonary (lung) involvement. Respiratory symptoms could range from a nagging dry cough and shortness of breath to more alarming symptoms like hemoptysis (coughing out blood).

Renal manifestations may remain subtler in the initial stages but can quickly escalate to more severe symptoms like foamy urine or even kidney failure in advanced cases.

In terms of diagnosis, radiological evaluation provides valuable insights into lung involvement, with chest X-rays or CT scans revealing possible lung hemorrhages. Along with radiology, blood tests for anti-glomerular basement membrane (anti-GBM) antibodies and kidney biopsies can confirm the diagnosis.

Treatment strategies for Goodpasture's syndrome hinge on dampening the rampant immune response and managing the organ-specific symptoms. This may involve the use of immunosuppressive agents along with plasmapheresis—a procedure that filters the anti-GBM antibodies out of the blood. For advanced cases with kidney failure, renal replacement therapy or kidney transplantation may be necessary.

Goodpasture's syndrome unfurls as a potent force in the realm of autoimmune disorders, necessitating swift recognition, decisive diagnostic drive, and intensive treatment approach for a favorable disease outcome.

Etiology and Epidemiology:

The exact cause of Goodpasture's syndrome is unknown, but it is believed to involve a combination of genetic and environmental factors. In this condition, the immune system produces antibodies that target a specific protein called collagen type IV, which is found in the basement membranes of the lungs and kidneys.

Goodpasture's syndrome is rare, with an estimated incidence of 0.5 to 1 case per million individuals per year. It primarily affects young adults, with a peak incidence in the third and fourth decades of life.

Clinical Symptoms:

The clinical presentation of Goodpasture's syndrome is characterized by respiratory and renal symptoms. Patients often experience cough, dyspnea (shortness of breath), hemoptysis (coughing up blood), and chest pain due to lung involvement. Renal symptoms may include hematuria (blood in the urine), proteinuria (protein in the urine), and decreased urine output.

Other systemic symptoms may include fatigue, weight loss, and joint pain. The severity of symptoms can vary, and prompt recognition is crucial for early intervention.

Radiological Evaluation:

Radiological evaluation, particularly high-resolution computed tomography (HRCT) scans, plays a significant role in assessing lung involvement in Goodpasture's syndrome. HRCT scans can reveal characteristic findings such as patchy ground-glass opacities, consolidations, and areas of hemorrhage in the lungs.

Renal imaging, such as ultrasound or computed tomography (CT), may be performed to evaluate kidney involvement and identify any structural abnormalities.

Treatment/Management:

When charting a course through the turbulent waves of Goodpasture's syndrome treatment, the primary objective is to rein in the overactive immune response, control the ensuing inflammation, and preserve the lungs and kidneys' function - the two main organs in the disease's firing line.

Doing so necessitates a therapeutic approach that blends immunosuppressive therapy, plasmapheresis, and supportive care into an efficient regimen.

Immunosuppressive medications like corticosteroids and cyclophosphamide form the backbone of therapy, aiming to suppress the immune system's production of harmful antibodies and dampen the overly exuberant immune response. The introduction of these agents helps to mitigate the ongoing attack on the body's tissues, making them invaluable in the early stages of the disease and allowing for control of active disease.

Alongside immunosuppression, plasma exchange emerges as a crucial player, especially when the disease presents aggressively or doesn't respond satisfactorily to medication alone.

This procedure, which mechanically filters the harmful anti-glomerular basement membrane (anti-GBM) antibodies from the blood, can rapidly reduce the levels of these pathogenic proteins and aid in curtailing the disease's immediate impact.

However, beyond these front-line interventions, the overall management of Goodpasture's syndrome entails an equally important layer of supportive care. As the disease wreaks havoc on the lungs and kidneys, supportive strategies like dialysis for renal failures or oxygen therapy for significant lung involvement may become necessary. Such measures help in symptom management, prevent or mitigate immediate complications, and sustain the patient's physiological balance during the disease's acute phase.

Moreover, an often-underestimated aspect of dealing with Goodpasture's syndrome is the need for diligent long-term follow-up and monitoring. Given the potential of disease relapse or long-term complications, regular monitoring helps ensure timely intervention and assists in maintaining the disease under long-term control.

Conclusion:

Goodpasture's syndrome exists as a rare but formidable representative of autoimmune diseases, distinguished by the paradox of the immune system launching an assault against the body's own lungs and kidneys. The complexity of this condition and its potential severity necessitates a fight on several fronts   early recognition, accurate diagnosis, immediate initiation of therapy, and long-term monitoring.

While the medical community has made significant strides in combating Goodpasture's syndrome, there remains an undeniable need for ongoing research. Enhancing our understanding of the disease's underlying mechanisms, honing in on the genetic and environmental triggers, and developing more effective, targeted therapies can revolutionize the approach to this challenging condition.

References:

1. Pusey CD. Anti-glomerular basement membrane disease. Lancet. 2003; 364(9457): 945-956.
2. Levy JB, Turner AN, Rees AJ, Pusey CD. Long-term outcome of anti-glomerular basement membrane antibody disease treated with plasma exchange and immunosuppression. Ann Intern Med. 2001; 134(11): 1033-1042.

"Cryptogenic Organizing Pneumonia (COP)": Inflammatory Lung Disease Leading to the Formation of Granulation Tissue and Organizing Pneumonia.

Sub-title: Inflammatory Lung Disease Leading to the Formation of Granulation Tissue and Organizing Pneumonia

Incidence: 1 to 2 people per 100,000
M/F: 1 / 1

Introduction:

Navigating the world of inflammatory lung diseases, Cryptogenic Organizing Pneumonia (COP), claiming its niche, emerges as a particularly intriguing entity. At its core, COP is symbolized by a rampant inflammation that sets the stage for the formation of granulation tissue—a kind of tissue generated in response to injury in the small airways and alveoli, the tiny air sacs deep within the lungs. This leads to a scenario of organizing pneumonia, a condition.

Navigating the intricate world of inflammatory lung diseases unveils Cryptogenic Organizing Pneumonia (COP)—a fascinating condition marked by relentless inflammation in the lungs, culminating in the formation of granulation tissue and the onset of organizing pneumonia.

This phenomenon essentially describes the lung's reaction to an injury or insult, unidentified in the case of COP, hence the term 'cryptogenic,' meaning 'of unknown origin.'

Etiology and Epidemiology:

The exact cause of COP is often unknown, hence the term "cryptogenic." However, it can be associated with various factors, including infections, drug reactions, connective tissue diseases, and inhalation exposures. The prevalence of COP is difficult to determine due to its underdiagnosis and variable clinical presentation. It can occur at any age but is more commonly observed in middle-aged and older adults.

Clinical Symptoms:

The clinical symptoms of COP are nonspecific and can mimic other respiratory conditions. Patients with COP may experience symptoms such as cough, dyspnea (shortness of breath), fatigue, and flu-like symptoms.

Some individuals may also have low-grade fever, weight loss, and chest discomfort.

The severity and duration of symptoms can vary, with some patients experiencing acute or subacute episodes and others having a more chronic course.

Radiological Evaluation:

Radiological evaluation, particularly high-resolution computed tomography (HRCT) scans, plays a crucial role in diagnosing and assessing the extent of lung involvement in COP. HRCT scans typically reveal patchy areas of ground-glass opacities, consolidations, and areas of bronchial wall thickening.

These findings are consistent with the presence of organizing pneumonia and can help differentiate COP from other interstitial lung diseases.

Treatment/Management:

Embarking on a strategic pathway for Cryptogenic Organizing Pneumonia's (COP) management underscores several key objectives—curtailing inflammation, fostering lung-tissue healing, and managing symptoms. Achieving these goals requires a broad therapeutic brush, the bristles of which are various medical and supportive interventions.

The mainstay for managing COP has traditionally been corticosteroids, such as prednisone. The potent anti-inflammatory abilities of these agents offer significant relief, leading to symptom reduction, and kickstarting the healing of lung tissues.

Given the chronicity of the inflammatory process in COP, these medications are often prescribed over an extensive duration, spanning several months at the least.

However, long-term use of corticosteroids manifold concerns, such as significant side effects and the potential development of steroid resistance. To mitigate these challenges, immunosuppressive agents come into the picture.

Medications like azathioprine and mycophenolate mofetil can prove potent comrades in COP's battle, as they can modulate the immune response and also assist in tapering the need for long-term corticosteroids use.

Often, strategies beyond medication become crucial components of COP's comprehensive management plan. For instance, supportive care can act as a linchpin, catering to managing symptoms and complications, and enhancing the overall treatment's effectiveness. Patients with significant respiratory discomfort may benefit from oxygen therapy, ensuring adequate oxygenation.

Conclusion:

In the chessboard of inflammatory lung diseases, Cryptogenic Organizing Pneumonia (COP) stands as an uncrowned rook. Primarily defined by the formation of granulation tissue and organizing pneumonia, COP largely remains idiopathic—its etiology veiled in obscurity.

In the chessboard of inflammatory lung diseases, Cryptogenic Organizing Pneumonia (COP) stands as an uncrowned rook. Primarily defined by the formation of granulation tissue and organizing pneumonia, COP largely remains idiopathic—its etiology veiled in obscurity.

From environmental factors to underlying immunological alterations, numerous theories shroud the enigma of the underlying cause, yet a definitive trigger eludes medical understanding.

At present, the cardinal strategy that propels effective patient management with COP revolves around early detection, precise diagnosis, and timely initiation of an individualized treatment regimen.

The goal revolves not only around symptom management and halting the disease's immediate progression but also in preserving lung function in the long term and minimizing the risk of relapse.

However, while current management protocols for COP can often control the condition effectively, complete cure remains elusive. A significant proportion of patients have recurrent disease or persistent lung abnormalities, underscoring the need for continued research in this area.

Moving forward, the field of COP requires profound research involvement—aimed at unearthing the latent etiological factors and understanding the underlying immune dysregulation mechanisms. Such knowledge could help fine-tune diagnostic protocols, aiding the clinical identification of potential risk factors and disease triggers.

Furthermore, insights into the disease's molecular and cellular underpinnings can guide the development of targeted therapies that address the root cause rather than merely controlling the symptoms.

Therefore, while we have made strides in managing COP, driving the prognosis from fatal to chronic over the last few decades, significant challenges persist.

Advancements in research to enhance the understanding of disease biology, development of effective therapeutic strategies, and improvement in supportive care are needed to unravel and address COP's cryptic nature, enabling clinicians to improve disease outcomes and patients' quality of life.

References:

1. Cordier JF. Cryptogenic organizing pneumonia. Clin Chest Med. 2004;25(4):727-738.
2. Drakopanagiotakis F, Paschalaki K, Abu-Hijleh M, et al. Cryptogenic and secondary organizing pneumonia: clinical presentation, radiographic findings, treatment response, and prognosis. Chest. 2011;139(4):893-900.

"Actinomycosis": A Bacterial Infection Usually Involving the Lungs and Causing the Formation of Abscesses and Hard Lumps.

Sub-title: A Bacterial Infection Usually Involving the Lungs and Causing the Formation of Abscesses and Hard Lumps

Incidence: 1 per 300,000 people.
M/F: 3 / 1

Introduction:

Navigating through the realm of rare infections, one encounters Actinomycosis—a distinct type of bacterial infection. This typically long-term condition is marked by the formation of pus-filled abscesses and hard, fibrous lumps, known technically as granulomas.

This unusual manifestation of disease gives actinomycosis its characteristic clinical pattern. Known to be caused by bacteria from the Actinomyces species, which are usually present in the mouth and gut, this infection can occasionally become pathogenic, especially when they gain dominance.

Etiology and Epidemiology:

Actinomycosis is caused by bacteria from the Actinomyces species, particularly Actinomyces israelii. These bacteria are normally present in the oral cavity, gastrointestinal tract, and female genital tract. Infection occurs when there is a breach in the mucosal barrier, allowing the bacteria to invade surrounding tissues.

The incidence of actinomycosis is relatively low, and it can affect individuals of any age. Certain risk factors, such as poor oral hygiene, dental procedures, immunosuppression, and underlying chronic diseases, may increase the likelihood of infection.

Clinical Symptoms:

The clinical presentation of actinomycosis can vary depending on the site of infection. In cases involving the lungs, common symptoms include cough, chest pain, fever, and weight loss. Patients may also experience difficulty breathing and coughing up blood.

Actinomycosis can also affect other areas of the body, such as the cervicofacial region, abdomen, and pelvis, leading to specific symptoms related to the affected site. The disease often progresses slowly and can be mistaken for other conditions, resulting in delayed diagnosis.

Radiological Evaluation:

Radiological evaluation, particularly computed tomography (CT) scans, plays a vital role in the diagnosis and assessment of actinomycosis. CT scans can reveal characteristic findings such as the presence of abscesses, thick-walled cavities, and inflammatory masses. These imaging findings, along with clinical and laboratory data, aid in differentiating actinomycosis from other infectious or neoplastic processes.

Treatment/Management:

The treatment of actinomycosis involves a combination of surgical intervention and antimicrobial therapy. Surgical drainage and debridement may be necessary to remove abscesses and infected tissues. Antimicrobial therapy with high-dose penicillin or amoxicillin is the mainstay of treatment, and the duration of therapy can range from several weeks to months.

In cases of penicillin allergy, alternative antibiotics such as clindamycin or doxycycline may be used. Close follow-up and monitoring are essential to assess treatment response and prevent recurrence.

In confronting actinomycosis, clinicians resort to a potent arsenal of interventions-textbook surgical management combined with meticulously planned antimicrobial therapy. The first line of defence rests upon surgical intervention where the primary aim is to evacuate abscesses and extricate infected tissues.

The actions range from simple drainage to more extensive debridement, dependent on disease extent, location, and individual patient factors. This surgery serves both to alleviate symptoms and to facilitate the impending medical management by reducing the disease burden.

Emerging next in the management pathway is an aggressive antimicrobial therapy. Here, robust antibiotics like high-dose penicillin or amoxicillin play a starring role. The robust antimicrobial action of these agents against the actin.

Conclusion:

In the maze of rare bacterial infections, Actinomycosis stands apart with its intricate pattern of abscess formation and hard lumps.

Even as a rarity, it emphasizes the essence of early recognition, precise diagnosis, and well-orchestrated management in the infectious disease arena. Undeniably, for those wading through the treacherous waters of actinomycosis, these factors can make a significant difference in disease outcomes.

However, to improve these very outcomes and to elevate the standard of patient care, the scientific community is called upon for further research. A deeper understanding of the underlying pathophysiology including the mechanisms of abscess formation and fibrosis, as well as colonization and invasion of actinomyces bacteria, could help us unearth modalities that offer not just treatment but also prevention of actinomycosis.

Moreover, optimizing current treatment strategies is a pressing requirement. Although medical management with anti-microbial therapy is usually effective, prolonged therapy timelines and the need for surgical intervention in many cases signal the necessity for more efficient, patient-friendly treatment options.

Understanding the disease better will allow us to tailor therapies, perhaps even on a personalized level based on patient characteristics, ensuring an optimal therapeutic response and minimizing burdens of treatment.

From an epidemiological perspective, identifying lifestyle, occupational, or geographical factors that might predispose individuals to actinomycosis may help understand disease patterns and develop preventive strategies. In a world where prevention often outweighs cure, formidable diseases like actinomycosis remind us of the importance of continuous learning, adaptation, and innovation.

To sum up, actinomycosis presents us with challenges of a rare, often insidious, yet decisively impactful disease. Navigating these challenges successfully demands a cohesive blend of early detection, accurate diagnostic ventures, appropriate therapeutic management, and crucially, continuous research aimed at understanding and addressing the disease's unique attributes.

Our battle against actinomycosis, though intricate, is far from insurmountable – every research stride brings us closer to better patient outcomes, bridging the gaps in our understanding and management of this distinctive disease.

References:
1. Valour F, Sénéchal A, Dupieux C, et al. Actinomycosis: etiology, clinical features, diagnosis, treatment, and management. Infect Drug Resist. 2014;7:183-197.
2. Smego RA Jr, Foglia G. Actinomycosis. Clin Infect Dis. 1998;26(6):1255-1261.

"Hypersensitivity Pneumonitis – HP": Understanding the Mechanisms, Clinical Presentation, and Management

Sub-Title: An In-Depth Analysis of Hypersensitivity Pneumonitis

Incidence: 0.4 to 7 per 100,000 people
M/F: 1 / 1

Introduction:

Hypersensitivity Pneumonitis (HP) is an immune-mediated lung disease characterized by inflammation in response to repeated exposure to environmental antigens. This article aims to provide a comprehensive understanding of HP, including its etiology, epidemiology, clinical symptoms, radiological evaluation, treatment, and management.

Traversing the intricate design of immune-mediated lung diseases, we encounter Hypersensitivity Pneumonitis (HP). This condition stands apart, owing to its unique mechanism—an inflammation-based response resulting from repeated exposure to certain environmental antigens.

The objective of this discussion is to present a thorough analysis of HP, examining its etiology, epidemiology, clinical manifestation, radiological evaluation, and potential treatment strategies.

Setting the stage for an in-depth understanding of HP, its etiology plays an instrumental role. The disease finds its genesis in an exaggerated immune response that the body mounts in the wake of repeated encounters with specific, often airborne

Etiology and Epidemiology:

HP is caused by an exaggerated immune response to inhaled organic or chemical antigens. The disease can be classified into three types based on the exposure source: bird-related, farmer's lung, and humidifier lung. HP can affect individuals of any age, gender, or ethnicity.

Certain occupations, such as farming, bird-keeping, and mold-exposed environments, have a higher risk of developing HP.

Clinical Symptoms:

The clinical presentation of HP can vary depending on the duration and intensity of antigen exposure. Common symptoms include cough, shortness of breath, chest tightness, and fatigue. Constitutional symptoms, such as fever and weight loss, may also be present. Symptoms typically occur a few hours after exposure and may resolve with avoidance of the antigen. If exposure continues, chronic HP can develop, leading to irreversible lung damage.

Radiological Evaluation:

Radiological evaluation plays a vital role in diagnosing HP. High-resolution computed tomography (HRCT) scans are the imaging modality of choice. HRCT findings typically show ground-glass opacities, centrilobular nodules, and air trapping. These findings, along with a compatible clinical history, are suggestive of HP.

Lung biopsies may be necessary in atypical cases or to confirm the diagnosis.

Treatment/Management:

When steering the treatment and management strategy for Hypersensitivity Pneumonitis (HP), the first and foremost principle hinges on avoidance of the offending antigen. A crucial step in this direction involves exhaustive efforts to identify potential sources of antigen exposure and systematically eliminating them, preventing repeat evocation of the immune response.

Emergencies or acute exacerbations may necessitate the use of corticosteroids—a potent class of anti-inflammatory drugs. These drugs hold authority over the inflammation that fuels HP's pathology.

Navigating the realm of Hypersensitivity Pneumonitis' (HP) treatment and management, the primary strategy unfurls in one simple yet fundamental mantra - avoidance of the causative antigen. This approach necessitates detailed exploration to identify the environmental sources triggering the antigen exposure, followed by diligently eliminating or at least minimizing these exposures.

This intuitive measure goes a long way in preventing fresh attacks of hypersensitivity responses and marks the first meaningful step towards arresting disease progression.

In the backdrop of acute exacerbations or when facing aggressive disease forms, corticosteroids become imperative in the therapeutic strategy. These powerful anti-inflammatory agents become a forth of defence against the rampant inflammation that propels HP's pathology, by dampening the exaggerated immune response.

However, the decision to embark on long-term corticosteroid therapy rides on a delicate balance. The risk of potential side effects - ranging from the metabolic, skeletal to even psychological disruptions - tethered to prolonged corticosteroid use should be kept in mind.

Conclusion:

Tucked within the library of immune-mediated lung diseases is Hypersensitivity Pneumonitis (HP)—a novel read concerning an overactive immune response to constant exposure to specific environmental antigens.

It becomes essential for clinicians to garner a comprehensive understanding of HP's highlights – the etiology that traces back to repeated antigen exposure, the clinical symptoms that unveil the body's rebellion against self, the radiological evaluations that provide a sneak peek into the lung's microscopic world, and management strategies furnishing a roadmap to recovery.

Grasping these chapters bolsters the currency needed for accurate diagnosis and effective treatment strategies.

Nestled within the compendium of immune-mediated lung diseases resides Hypersensitivity Pneumonitis (HP)—a remarkable narrative about an overactive immune response provoked by recurrent environmental antigen exposure.

As clinicians and medical researchers, it becomes critical to sift through and thoroughly understand the various layers of HP, including the etiology, symptoms, radiological evaluation, and possible intervention strategies. Such an understanding forms the foundation of targeted diagnostic processes and enables the formulation of effective treatment modalities.

Emerging as the key protagonist in managing HP is avoidance—a practice centered on the identification and subsequent elimination of exposure to the offending antigen. This crucial step not only stands as a preventive measure but also acts as the first strike against the disease's progression.

In instances of acute HP episodes or flare-ups, corticosteroids, potent anti-inflammatory allies, step into the fray. They work to douse the flames of inflammation – a hallmark of HP – thereby providing immediate relief.

However, this alliance must be cautiously drawn, keeping in mind the potential side-effects that escort prolonged corticosteroid usage.

References:
1. Selman M, et al. Hypersensitivity pneumonitis: a multifaceted deceiving disorder. Seminars in Respiratory and Critical Care Medicine. 2012;33(5):519-531.
2. Lacasse Y, et al. Clinical presentation, investigation, and management of hypersensitivity pneumonitis. Expert Review of Respiratory Medicine. 2016;10(11):1185-1203.
3. Vourlekis JS, et al. Hypersensitivity pneumonitis. Clinical Reviews in Allergy & Immunology. 2003;24(2):103-132.

"Eosinophilic Granuloma - EG": A Rare Condition Characterized by Eosinophil Infiltration and Lung Inflammation.

Sub-title: A Rare Condition Characterized by Eosinophil Infiltration and Lung Inflammation

Incidence: 1 to 2 adults per million
M/F: 1 / 1

Introduction

In the realm of infrequent conditions, Eosinophilic Granuloma emerges as a medical marvel, distinguished by eosinophil infiltration inducing lung inflammation. Eosinophils constitute a sub-section of the body's white blood cells that usually target and combat parasitic infections.

In Eosinophilic Granuloma, however, these immune cells see an unusual build-up, particularly in the lung tissues, setting the stage for inflammation.

Interestingly, Eosinophilic Granuloma is not a stand-alone entity but is considered a localized representation of a wider spectrum of diseases known as Langerhans Cell Histiocytosis (LCH). The LCH family comprises disorders unified by the abnormal proliferation of Langerhans cells—immune cells involved in presenting foreign substances to the immune system—in different body organs.

However, in Eosinophilic Granuloma, the predominant involvement is the lungs, setting the foundation for unique clinical and radiological features associated with this disease.

If we delve deeper into the etiology of Eosinophilic Granuloma, we encounter an interesting tie between genetic components and potential environmental triggers such as smoking. However, understanding this riddle of causation still remains fledgling, necessitating further research.

From an epidemiological standpoint, Eosinophilic Granuloma is a rarity. Nevertheless, its incidence is slightly greater in smokers and in males, with the disease often manifesting in young adulthood.

Clinically, Eosinophilic Granuloma paints a diverse picture. Some patients may be completely asymptomatic, with the condition picked up incidentally on imaging studies. Others, however, could present with a range of respiratory complaints, such as cough, chest pain, and potentially more severe manifestations like breathing difficulties or even lung collapse in advanced cases.

Diagnosis of Eosinophilic Granuloma unifies clinical evaluation, radiological findings, and sometimes, biopsy results. Imaging techniques like chest X-ray or CT scans can reveal classic signs like cystic changes or "punched-out" lesions. However, a definitive diagnosis often relies on a lung biopsy, revealing characteristic findings of eosinophilic infiltration and abnormal Langerhans cells.

Etiology and Epidemiology:

The exact cause of Eosinophilic Granuloma is unknown, but it is believed to result from an abnormal immune response. It primarily affects children and young adults, with a slight male predominance. The condition is rare, accounting for approximately 10% of all LCH cases.

Clinical Symptoms:

Patients with Eosinophilic Granuloma often present with nonspecific symptoms such as cough, chest pain, and shortness of breath. These symptoms may be attributed to the inflammation and mass effect caused by the eosinophilic infiltrate.

Systemic symptoms like fever and weight loss are less common in Eosinophilic Granuloma compared to other forms of LCH.

Radiological Evaluation:

Radiological evaluation plays a crucial role in the diagnosis of Eosinophilic Granuloma. Chest X-rays may reveal solitary or multiple pulmonary nodules, which are often well-defined and may have a characteristic "punched out" appearance.

Computed Tomography (CT) scans provide more detailed information about the extent of lung involvement and aid in differentiating Eosinophilic Granuloma from other lung diseases.

Treatment/Management:

The pathway to Eosinophilic Granuloma's management charts its course based on several variables—the extent of the disease, current respiratory function, and the patient's general health status.

For patients who harbor a localized form of the disease and grapple with minimal symptoms, a conservative management strategy may suffice.

Such management relies on regular monitoring rather than aggressive intervention. It includes regular health check-ups focusing on the clinical evolution of the condition, and radiological assessments to evaluate the disease's progression or stability over time.

The ultimate aim with this approach is to delay or potentially avoid the need for more intensive treatment options, particularly given the potential side-effects associated with these.

However, as the disease discourse changes—marked by an escalation of symptoms, more widespread lung involvement, or development of complications—a less complacent approach is needed. Here, systemic therapies mark the preferred choice, varying from corticosteroid therapy or potentially chemotherapy agents in severe cases.

Corticosteroids, owing to their potent anti-inflammatory effects, can help combat the inflammation imbued by eosinophil build-up, thereby providing symptomatic relief and arresting further inflammatory damage. However, their long-term usage warrants caution due to their side effect profile.

For patients with severely symptomatic, progressive, or corticosteroid-refractory Eosinophilic Granuloma, chemotherapy emerges as a potential option. Medications like vinblastine or methotrexate, initially developed for managing malignancies, have now found their place in the repertoire of management strategies for Eosinophilic Granuloma.

These agents work by combatting the abnormal proliferation of Langerhans cells, thereby halting the disease process. However, the benefits of chemotherapy should be weighed against its potential side effects, including increased infection susceptibility or organ toxicities.

Regardless of the chosen management strategy, all patients with Eosinophilic Granuloma should be closely monitored to evaluate the treatment's effectiveness, gauge disease progression, and ensure timely intervention in the face of potential complications.

To sum up, Eosinophilic Granuloma, although a relatively rare cause of lung disease, presents a noteworthy challenge due to its potentially progressive nature, complex diagnostics, and intricate management strategies.

Striding ahead, it becomes essential to further research in understanding the disease's basic mechanisms and improving diagnostic and treatment approaches, aiming to improvise patient outcomes.

Global collaboration and multi-disciplinary approaches will be invaluable tools in our ongoing journey to decrypt this complex entity.

Conclusion:

Eosinophilic Granuloma is a rare condition characterized by the infiltration of eosinophils, leading to lung inflammation. Although it is a localized form of LCH, its clinical presentation, radiological features, and management differ from other LCH variants. Early diagnosis and appropriate management are crucial to minimize complications and improve outcomes for affected individuals.

In the sprawling world of rare pulmonary conditions, Eosinophilic Granuloma carves a unique niche, characterized by a peculiar infiltration of eosinophils and leading to lung inflammation.

Though it resides under the umbrella of Langerhans Cell Histiocytosis (LCH), it firmly holds its ground with distinguishable clinical presentations, radiological features, and management strategies, setting it apart from other LCH variants.

Eosinophilic Granuloma tells a compelling tale of the body's fascinating immune response. An otherwise beneficial immune element—the eosinophils—becomes the harbinger of disease due to an excessive build-up and infiltration in the lung tissue, leading to localized inflammation and granuloma formation.

The disease's nebulous presentation ranges from minimal symptoms to severe respiratory distress, cementing the importance of a high index of suspicion and meticulous evaluation in its identification. Its radiological persona often reflects classic manifestations like cystic changes or "punched-out" lesions.

References:

1. Vassallo R. Eosinophilic lung diseases: diagnostic challenges and therapeutic options. Expert Rev Respir Med. 2017;11(6):425-434.
2. Chuang CC, et al. Eosinophilic lung diseases: a clinical, radiologic, and pathologic overview. Radiographics. 2014;34(3):e43-e56.

"Berylliosis": A Lung Disease Caused by Beryllium Exposure, Resulting in Granuloma Formation.

Sub-title: "Industrial Enemy: Berylliosis – The Hidden Hazards of Beryllium Exposure to the Lungs"

Incidence: Not well established
M/F: Male-dominant

Introduction

In the array of occupational lung diseases, Berylliosis shines its spotlight. At its core, it is an inflammatory reaction ignited by exposure to beryllium—a lightweight metal frequently employed in a plethora of industries, including the aerospace domain, electronics industries, and nuclear power facilities. Inhalation of beryllium particles acts as the catalyst that sets off an immune response that ultimately manifests as the formation of granulomas in the lungs.

At the heart of Berylliosis's development is the role of beryllium. As a metal, it poses no threat; however, when it enters the lungs in the form of dust or fumes—the likelihood in industrial settings—things take a grim turn. Beryllium particles, once in the body, can trigger an immune response.

The immune system, in an attempt to contain these foreign bodies, leads to the formation of granulomas—a kind of tissue inflammation characterized by the accumulation of immune cells.

The likelihood of Berylliosis is closely linked to occupational exposure—people working in industries where beryllium is processed or manufactured stand at higher risk. However, even within this risk population, certain genetic predispositions might amplify the chances of developing berylliosis, thus adding a layer of complexity in delineating the true etiology of this condition.

Epidemiologically, while Berylliosis is relatively rare in the general population, it gains significance in workers exposed to beryllium. Efforts to curb occupational exposure to beryllium dust and fumes are therefore crucial in controlling the disease's incidence.

Clinically, like many other lung diseases, Berylliosis brandishes a spectrum of respiratory symptoms. Cough, chest pain, shortness of breath—all varying in severity—are typical call signs of Berylliosis.

More severe forms of the disease might include weight loss, fatigue, and night sweats.

Etiology and Epidemiology:

Beryllium, in its various forms, can induce an exaggerated immune response in susceptible individuals. The exact mechanisms underlying the development of berylliosis are not fully understood, but it is believed to involve a combination of genetic and environmental factors.

Berylliosis is an occupationally acquired disease, primarily affecting workers exposed to beryllium dust, fumes, or other forms of the metal. The incidence of berylliosis varies among different industries and geographical regions.

Clinical Symptoms:

The symptoms of berylliosis can range from mild to severe, depending on the extent and duration of exposure. Acute berylliosis typically presents with flu-like symptoms, including fever, fatigue, cough, and shortness of breath.

Chronic berylliosis, which develops after prolonged exposure, may manifest as progressive dyspnea, chest pain, and weight loss. In some cases, berylliosis can also affect other organs, leading to skin rashes, joint pain, and liver abnormalities.

Radiological Evaluation:

Radiological evaluation plays a crucial role in the diagnosis and monitoring of berylliosis. Chest X-rays and high-resolution computed tomography (HRCT) scans are commonly used to assess lung involvement.

These imaging techniques can reveal characteristic findings such as bilateral micronodular opacities, hilar lymphadenopathy, and interstitial lung disease. The presence of granulomas, although not specific to berylliosis, can provide supportive evidence for the diagnosis.

Treatment/Management:

In a disease like Berylliosis, where certain environmental exposure forms the cornerstone of its pathogenesis, management strategies naturally pivot on eliminating this exposure. The first checkpoint on this management pathway is preventing further exposure to beryllium.

Achieving this demands implementing a seamless blend of engineering controls to reduce ambient levels of beryllium in workplaces, wearing personal protective equipment to minimize individual exposure, and stringent adherence to occupational safety rules and guidelines.

However, managing Berylliosis is not limited to exposure precautions. When symptoms make their mark, medical management comes into the frame. Corticosteroids become the front-line pharmacological agents due to their potent anti-inflammatory properties, helping subvert the immune overreaction that paves the way for granuloma formation in Berylliosis.

But corticosteroid therapy, though effective, may not prove sufficient for all, particularly those with severe or refractory disease. Here, a more aggressive form of therapy—immunosuppressive agents—may be required. Medications such as methotrexate or azathioprine can help thwart the exaggerated immune response, offering a potential shot at symptom control and disease management.

To ensure the chosen treatment approach is hitting its intended mark, and also to keep an eye on the disease's potential progression, regular monitoring becomes essential. This includes periodic lung function tests to assess respiratory performance and radiological evaluations to visualize any alterations in lung structure or detect early signs of complications.

In conclusion, managing Berylliosis demands a robust approach—one that not only addresses the disease's underlying cause but also its symptomatic manifestations, while concurrently monitoring disease trajectory. It is a delicate balancing act, ensuring optimal patient outcomes while minimizing exposure to potential side-effects of therapy.

Conclusion:

Berylliosis is a lung disease caused by exposure to beryllium, leading to the formation of granulomas in the lungs. Occupational exposure is the primary route of acquisition, and early recognition is crucial to prevent disease progression. A comprehensive approach involving prevention, prompt diagnosis, and appropriate management is essential to minimize the impact of berylliosis on affected individuals.

Among the diaspora of occupational lung diseases, Berylliosis stakes its claim as a condition driven by exposure to beryllium and characterized by an inflammatory response that culminates in the formation of granulomas in the lungs.

Occupations that deal with beryllium processing or manufacturing transform into the focal point for berylliosis, marking occupational exposure as the principal route of acquisition.

Recognizing this disease early in its course presents a significant advantage, setting the foundation for timely intervention and preventing disease progression. It necessitates vigilance on the part of healthcare professionals, particularly those involved in occupational health and safety, to promptly identify potential cases based on risk factors and symptomatology.

Management of Berylliosis requires a comprehensive and strategic approach—one that seamlessly weaves together the threads of prevention, diagnostics, and therapeutics to construct a united front against the disease. It starts with preventive measures, focusing on minimizing beryllium exposure in workplace settings through engineering controls, personal protective equipment, and strict adherence to safety guidelines.

References:

1. Newman LS, Maier LA. Beryllium disease. Lung. 1999;177(6):363-388.
2. Henneberger PK, et al. Beryllium sensitization and disease among long-term and short-term workers in a beryllium ceramics plant. Int Arch Occup Environ Health. 2001;74(3):167-176.
3. Rossman MD, et al. The beryllium lymphocyte proliferation test: relevant issues in beryllium health surveillance. Am J Ind Med. 1997;32(4):337-340.

"Pulmonary Alveolar Microlithiasis (PAM)": A Genetic Disorder Characterized by Alveolar Calcium Phosphate Microlith Accumulation

Sub-title: "Pulmonary Alveolar Microlithiasis (PAM)": A Genetic Disorder Characterized by Alveolar Calcium Phosphate Microlith Accumulation

Incidence: 1,300 cases since 1918
M/F: 1 / 1

Introduction:

Pulmonary Alveolar Microlithiasis (PAM) is a rare genetic disorder characterized by the abnormal accumulation of calcium phosphate microliths in the alveoli of the lungs. This article provides an overview of PAM, including its etiology, epidemiology, clinical symptoms, radiological evaluation, treatment, and management.

Just off the beaten path of common pulmonary conditions, Pulmonary Alveolar Microlithiasis (PAM) takes root. It's a moniker that might sound like a mouthful, but disassembled, it demystifies the rare genetic disorder at hand. 'Pulmonary' and 'alveolar' gesture towards the disease's preferred site—the lungs, more specifically, the tiny air sacs or alveoli within them. 'Microlithiasis' reveals the guest of concern—minuscule stones, or microliths, composed of calcium phosphate.

Delving into PAM's etiology unveils a noteworthy facet—it's a disorder with a genetic underpinning. More precisely, mutations in the SLC34A2 gene—encoding a protein involved in phosphate transport—are usually the culprits behind this disorder. These mutations disrupt normal phosphate transport and lead to phosphate build-up in the lungs, triggering the production of calcium phosphate microliths that deposit in the alveoli.

Etiology and Epidemiology:

PAM is primarily caused by mutations in the SLC34A2 gene, which encodes the sodium-phosphate cotransporter type 2b (NPT2b) protein. The exact mechanisms through which these mutations lead to microlith formation are not fully understood.

PAM is inherited in an autosomal recessive manner, and consanguinity in affected families is common. The disorder has been reported worldwide, but its prevalence varies among different populations.

Clinical Symptoms:

PAM is often asymptomatic in the early stages, and diagnosis is frequently incidental. However, as the disease progresses, clinical manifestations may develop. Common symptoms include progressive dyspnea, cough, chest pain, and fatigue.

Some individuals may experience recurrent respiratory infections or hemoptysis. In severe cases, PAM can lead to respiratory failure and pulmonary hypertension, significantly impacting the patient's quality of life.

Radiological Evaluation:

Radiological evaluation plays a critical role in the diagnosis of PAM. Chest X-rays typically show diffuse, bilateral, and symmetric nodular opacities, which resemble a "sandstorm" pattern.

High-resolution computed tomography (HRCT) scans provide more detailed information and can reveal the characteristic findings of numerous, tiny, and calcified micronodules diffusely distributed throughout the lung parenchyma. Lung biopsies are rarely necessary for diagnosis but may be considered in atypical cases.

Treatment/Management:

Currently, there is no specific cure for PAM. The management of this condition primarily focuses on symptomatic relief and prevention of complications. Regular monitoring of lung function and radiological assessments is essential to assess disease progression.

Symptomatic treatment includes bronchodilators, inhaled corticosteroids, and antibiotics for respiratory infections. Lung transplantation may be considered in severe cases of respiratory failure.

At present, our medical orchestra doesn't play a curative tune for Pulmonary Alveolar Microlithiasis (PAM). Instead, the approach skirts around the edges, primarily focusing on providing symptomatic relief, preventing or managing complications, and monitoring disease progression.

Regular assessment of lung function is critical, using tools such as pulmonary function tests that offer valuable insights into lung capacity and function.

In the realm of Pulmonary Alveolar Microlithiasis (PAM), the wave of a magic curative wand does not exist. Instead, our toolbox contains a strategic approach primarily aimed at symptom relief, staving off complications, and keeping a close eye to monitor any shifts in the disease's trajectory.

Regular health assessments lie at the heart of this management strategy. Evaluating lung function periodically forms a crucial component and utilizes tools such as spirometry.

Conclusion:

Taking a walk in the park of rare genetic disorders, one might stumble upon Pulmonary Alveolar Microlithiasis (PAM)—an unusual condition distinguished by the abnormal build-up of calcium phosphate microliths within the alveoli of the lungs. The root cause of this specific disorder points towards certain mutations in the 'SLC34A2' gene.

These genetic anomalies disrupt the normal functionality of the gene product responsible for phosphate transport, ultimately leading to phosphate accumulation in the lungs and the formation of calcium phosphate microliths.

Beyond its unique genetic predisposition, PAM delves into an interesting plethora of clinical manifestations. Hyphenating the spectrum between asymptomatic individuals to those crippled by pulmonary dysfunction, this ailment affirms the importance of comprehensive clinical evaluation and radiological imaging in piecing together a diagnosis.

Radiological evaluation plays a significant role in this process. A classic 'sandstorm' pattern emerging on chest X-rays or high-resolution CT scan can offer diagnostic clues. However, definitiveness may require a lung biopsy demonstrating characteristic alveolar microliths, though this more invasive method is reserved for cases where diagnosis is otherwise unclear.

Despite advances in medical genetics and therapeutics, PAM continues to be an incurable condition. Yet, a beacon of hope shines upon management strategies aimed at symptom alleviation and complication prevention.

At present, symptomatic management reigns as a key player in PHM's care algorithm. Bronchodilators play a role in patients with bronchospasm or obstructive ventilatory defects, whereas inhaled corticosteroids are used in patients with an inflammatory phenotype. Despite these therapies' effectiveness, they help manage the disease rather than erase its existence.

For severe cases or those marked by life-threatening respiratory failure,

References:

1. Castellana G, et al. Pulmonary alveolar microlithiasis: clinical features, evolution of the phenotype, and review of the literature. Am J Respir Crit Care Med. 2006;174(8):810-816.
2. Huqun, et al. Mutations in the SLC34A2 gene are associated with pulmonary alveolar microlithiasis. Am J Respir Crit Care Med. 2007;175(3):263-268.
3. Mariotta S, et al. Pulmonary alveolar microlithiasis: report on 576 cases published in the literature. Sarcoidosis Vasc Diffuse Lung Dis. 2004;21(3):173-181.

"Lymphocytic Interstitial Pneumonia (LIP)": A rare condition involving the infiltration of lymphocytes into the lung tissue, causing inflammation.

Sub-Title: Unpacking the Unique Characteristics and Management Strategies for LIP

Incidence: A few hundred cases have been reported
M/F: 1 / 2 and 1 / 3

Introduction

Lymphocytic interstitial pneumonia (LIP) is a relatively uncommon condition primarily affecting the lungs. This disorder is uniquely characterized by the infiltration of immune cells known as lymphocytes into the lung tissue, creating inflammation. Lymphocytes, a type of white blood cell, play a crucial role in the body's immune response. Yet, when they infiltrate the delicate lung tissue and incite an inflammatory response, they can lead to severe and potentially devastating health issues like LIP.

Although LIP is not a well-known condition due to its rarity, it remains an essential part of the larger landscape of pulmonary disorders, particularly those classified as interstitial lung diseases (ILDs). ILDs represent a collection of various lung disorders that are distinguished by their shared propensity for resulting in notable infiltration and inflammation of the lung's interstitial tissue.

When the intricate web of tissue and spaces around the alveoli—or tiny air sacs within the lungs—becomes inflamed or damaged, it can lead to a wide array of breathing problems and other respiratory symptoms. Among the numerous types of ILDs, LIP holds a unique place due to the involvement of lymphocytes.

Despite its rarity, LIP is more than just one of many obscure medical conditions. Detailed knowledge about this disorder holds high significance among healthcare providers, primarily because of its profound impact on those affected by it. The disease, like many ILDs, often carries a significant burden of symptoms.

These can include difficulty breathing, fatigue, and other problems that can substantially decrease a patient's quality of life. Furthermore, the potential progression of LIP from a manageable condition to a severe, life-threatening disease underlines the necessity of understanding this disease thoroughly.

For instance, in some cases, LIP can unexpectedly evolve into a lethally aggressive variety of lymphoma — a cancer of the lymphocytes that initially set the stage for LIP. This potential for progression to a more severe disease state—combined with the significant impact of LIP's symptoms on those who live with the condition—makes it clear that understanding of this disease is not a matter of academic interest alone.

Rather, it is a deeply impactful health issue that requires continued exploration and research to improve the lives of patients around the world who suffer from it.

Tos um up, despite the rarity of Lymphocytic Interstitial Pneumonia (LIP), it represents a significant health challenge that requires public awareness and dedicated research. By increasing our understanding of this disease's pathophysiology and clinical impact, we can create more effective strategies for treatment and, ultimately, prevention.

Etiology and Epidemiology

The exact cause of LIP is unknown but is believed to be associated with autoimmune or post-viral inflammatory responses. The disease has also been linked with certain other conditions, including Sjogren's syndrome, HIV infection, and primary immune disorders. LIP predominantly affects adults in their sixth decade of life, with a slight female preponderance. However, it can occur in patients of any age, including children.

Clinical symptoms

LIP symptomatology is non-specific, mainly characterized by dyspnea, non-productive cough, and generalized systemic symptoms such as fatigue and weight loss. More severe manifestations such as hemoptysis and chest pain can also occur in some patients.

Radiological evaluation

High-resolution computed tomography (HRCT) is a crucial tool for the radiological evaluation of LIP. The predominant radiologic appearances are ground-glass opacification, multiple thin-walled cysts, and diffuse nodules or reticular abnormalities across both lungs.

Treatment / Management

The mainstay of treatment and management for LIP hinges on corticosteroid therapy. Corticosteroids, a class of medication frequently utilized for their powerful anti-inflammatory properties, are primarily employed to reduce inflammation within the lungs. The goal of this treatment approach is twofold — first to alleviate the patient's symptomatic respiratory distress and secondly to abate the underlying pathologic inflammation spurring on the disease process.

While the deployed corticosteroid regimen may improve symptoms, it is typically a chronic management strategy intended to provide symptom control rather than cure.

Apart from pharmacological interventions, a spectrum of non-pharmacological techniques often complement the LIP management. One such is oxygen supplementation, which is particularly beneficial for patients exhibiting signs of respiratory distress or those with decreased oxygen saturation levels.

Oxygen supplementation aims to boost the oxygen levels within the patient's blood, thus assuaging the symptoms of respiratory distress and improving overall patient comfort.

Pulmonary rehabilitation, another key component of the disease management process, is a thorough, personalized program intended to enhance the patient's physical conditioning, disease knowledge, and self-management skills. This systematic and all-encompassing interventional strategy aims to improve the patient's overall health status and quality of life.

Among the spectrum of available treatment options, lung transplantation stands as the last resort, only considered in the most severe and life-threatening cases of LIP where all other treatment modalities fail to provide any significant progress.

Conclusion

In conclusion, Lymphocytic Interstitial Pneumonia (LIP) is a rare pulmonary disorder that necessitates due recognition for its potential clinical severity that penetrates deeply into the fine tissues that make up the lung's structure. It originates from a complex interplay between the lymphocytes and the lung tissue, leading to a characteristic infiltration and subsequent inflammation of lung tissues.

Delving deeper into the disease's etiology, understanding its varied clinical features, and harnessing the most effective strategies for its management emerge as the pillars for dealing optimally with LIP.

As we enhance our knowledge in these fields, we concurrently shore up our ability to manage patients suffering from this condition more successfully.

By improving our understanding not only of LIP but of the broader spectrum of interstitial lung diseases, we stand a much better chance of providing comprehensive care to the patients affected and continually improving their treatment outcomes.

Ultimately, the quest for improved management approaches for LIP underscores our broader mission in healthcare — to continually improve the lives of patients by developing a deeper understanding of diseases and establishing more effective strategies for their treatment and prevention.

References

1. Ryu, J.H., Myers, J.L., & Swensen, S.J. (2005). Diffuse Parenchymal Lung Disease: A Practical Approach. Mayo Clinic Proceedings, 80(4), 527-539.

2. Swigris, J.J., & Brown, K.K. (2010). Management of ILD-associated Cough. Chest, 138(1), 188-196.

3. Travis, W.D., Costabel, U., Hansell, D.M., et al. (2013). An Official American Thoracic Society/European Respiratory Society Statement: Update of the International Multidisciplinary Classification of the Idiopathic Interstitial Pneumonias. American Journal of Respiratory and Critical Care Medicine, 188(6), 733-748.

"Lymphocytic Bronchiolitis: Inflammatory Lung Disease Characterized by Lymphocytic Infiltration in the Bronchioles

Sub-Title: Understanding the Pathogenesis, Clinical Presentation, and Management of Lymphocytic Bronchiolitis

Incidence: Up to 50% of cases post-transplantation
M/F: is not specifically defined

Introduction:

Diving into the territory of inflammatory lung diseases, an encounter with Lymphocytic Bronchiolitis is inevitable. This illness presents a unique profile, featuring a targeted infiltration of lymphocytes—a type of white blood cell—into the bronchioles, the smaller passageways for air in the lungs.

This manuscript aims to illuminate the dark corners of Lymphocytic Bronchiolitis by expounding on its etiology, epidemiology, clinical presentation Extended Paragraph:

Venturing into the realm of inflammatory lung diseases unearths an intriguing entity known as Lymphocytic Bronchiolitis. This condition stands tall, etched by the characteristic infiltration of lymphocytes—immune cells integral to the body's defensive mechanism—into the bronchioles, the delicate airways in the lungs.

In this detailed exploration, we aim to disentangle the complex tapestry of Lymphocytic Bronchiolitis, encompassing its causes, epidemiological trends, clinical manifestations, radiological indicators, therapeutic interventions, and overarching management strategies.

Diving into the root causes of Lymphocytic Bronchiolitis uncovers a mix of intricately interwoven factors. Its primary characterization—the lymphocytic infiltration—is a telltale sign of the immune system at play. Affected individuals often have an underlying trigger, such as respiratory infections or exposures to irritants, which set the immune system into hyperdrive.

Etiology and Epidemiology:

The exact etiology of Lymphocytic Bronchiolitis is currently unknown. It is believed to involve an immune-mediated response triggered by various environmental factors, including viral infections, medications, and connective tissue diseases.

Lymphocytic Bronchiolitis is more commonly observed in middle-aged adults, with a higher prevalence in females. It can occur in isolation or in association with other lung diseases such as asthma or chronic obstructive pulmonary disease (COPD).

Clinical Symptoms:

The clinical presentation of Lymphocytic Bronchiolitis can vary widely. Common symptoms include persistent cough, shortness of breath, wheezing, and chest tightness. Some individuals may experience recurrent respiratory infections or have symptoms that mimic asthma exacerbations. In severe cases, respiratory failure may occur.

The disease progression and severity can vary among individuals, leading to a broad range of clinical manifestations.

Radiological Evaluation:

Radiological evaluation plays a crucial role in diagnosing Lymphocytic Bronchiolitis. High-resolution computed tomography (HRCT) scans are the imaging modality of choice.

HRCT findings typically show air trapping, bronchial wall thickening, and mosaic attenuation. These findings are indicative of small airway disease and can help differentiate Lymphocytic Bronchiolitis from other lung diseases with similar clinical presentations.

Treatment/Management:

The primary objective in the management of Lymphocytic Bronchiolitis is to minimize inflammation and relieve any discomforting symptoms that are associated with this respiratory condition. To control the inflammation in the airways, inhaled corticosteroids are frequently prescribed. These medications are designed to decrease swelling and irritation in the air passageways, thus bringing considerable relief to the patient.

Another set of medicines involved in the treatment strategy includes bronchodilators. These drugs are particularly useful in providing relief from bronchospasm, a condition characterized by abnormal constriction of the bronchial tubes.

Bronchodilators work by relaxing the muscles around the airways, thus widening them and improving the airflow to the lungs.

However, in severe cases, where patients fail to respond adequately to conventional therapy, the healthcare provider may consider prescribing immunosuppressive medications.

Treatments may include such drugs as azathioprine or mycophenolate mofetil. These medications are known to reduce immune system activity, thereby inducing a reduction in the inflammation of airways. However, they should be taken under strict medical supervision due to potential side effects.

To ensure effective management and control of this disease, the importance of regular follow-up visits with the healthcare provider cannot be overstated. These visits allow for close monitoring of the disease progression.

Moreover, it provides an opportunity for the healthcare provider to make necessary adjustments to the ongoing treatment plan as per the changing condition of the patient. This step is crucial in maximizing the effectiveness of the treatment protocol and ensuring an optimal quality of life for the patient.

Conclusion:

Lymphocytic Bronchiolitis, an inflammatory affliction identified predominantly in the lungs, is defined mainly by the infiltration of lymphocytes in bronchioles, those tiny air passages that substantiate the respiratory system.

Despite extensive studies and continuous research, the precise causative factor or the exact etiology continues to remain elusive. However, a possibility of an immune-mediated response acting as a crucial component in the disease's onset and progression has been theorized and widely accepted in the medical community.

Clinical manifestations of Lymphocytic Bronchiolitis are diverse and can vary considerably from one individual to another. They can range from mild respiratory distress to severe breathlessness, making it a challenging task to diagnose based on symptoms alone.

Hence, the role of radiological evaluation becomes incredibly significant. Tools such as computed tomography (CT) scans and chest x-rays aid in refining diagnosis accuracy, which is critical for devising an appropriate treatment plan.

While it's true that a definitive cure for Lymphocytic Bronchiolitis is yet to be discovered, it's crucial to remember that there are effective management strategies available. These strategies, primarily involving the use of corticosteroids, bronchodilators, and under certain circumstances, immune-suppressors, are integral to symptom relief.

The aim of these strategies is not only to regulate the inflammation and manage the breathing difficulties but to significantly enhance the quality of life for those diagnosed with the disease. In conclusion, the constantly improving understanding of Lymphocytic Bronchiolitis—along with its effective management protocols— offer substantial next steps in alleviating the affliction and fostering an improved quality of life for patients.

References:
1. Nicholson AG, et al. Lymphocytic bronchiolitis: an interstitial lung disease? Histopathology. 2002;41(4):313-322.
2. Travis WD, et al. Lymphoid hyperplasia and lymphocytic bronchiolitis. Seminars in Diagnostic Pathology. 1992;9(2):92-101.
3. Ryu JH, et al. Lymphocytic bronchiolitis/bronchitis. Seminars in Respiratory and Critical Care Medicine. 2003;24(5):461-467.

"Desquamative Interstitial Pneumonia (DIP): A Form of Interstitial Lung Disease Characterized by Alveolar Macrophage Accumulation

Sub-Title: Unraveling the Pathogenesis, Clinical Presentation, and Management of DIP

Incidence: Less than 1-2% of all interstitial lung disease cases
M/F: The actual ratio can vary

Introduction:

Belonging to the broad category of interstitial lung diseases, Desquamative Interstitial Pneumonia (DIP) presents a unique pathology characterized predominantly by the accumulation of macrophages within the alveoli - tiny air-filled sacs integral to the process of respiration.

This comprehensive discussion aims to delve deeper into understanding the many aspects of DIP, expanding upon its root causes (etiology), observable manifestations (clinical symptoms), and its incidence and distribution (epidemiology), all contributing to a holistic picture of the disease.

Further, crucial diagnostic tools, particularly the role of radiological evaluation in DIP, will be discussed in detail to provide an understanding of how internal structures of the lungs affected by DIP are examined and used to confirm diagnosis.

This article also intends to explore various treatment options and strategic management methods available for DIP, shedding light on the potential shifts in therapeutic approaches and providing approaches to handle this specific lung condition.

Through this, the piece aims to comprehensively dissect and present every aspect of DIP, thereby providing the reader a detailed understanding of this particular form of interstitial lung disease.

Etiology and Epidemiology:

The exact etiology of DIP is unknown; however, it is believed to be related to smoking and exposure to environmental factors. DIP is more commonly observed in individuals between the ages of 30 and 50, with a higher prevalence in males. It is often associated with a history of smoking and is considered a smoking-related interstitial lung disease.

Clinical Symptoms:

The clinical presentation of DIP is variable, with symptoms ranging from mild to severe. Common symptoms include progressive dyspnea, cough, and fatigue. Some individuals may experience weight loss and chest discomfort. In severe cases, respiratory failure may occur. Clinical manifestations may overlap with other interstitial lung diseases, making an accurate diagnosis crucial for appropriate management.

Radiological Evaluation:

Radiological evaluation plays a significant role in diagnosing DIP. High-resolution computed tomography (HRCT) scans are the imaging modality of choice. HRCT findings typically show ground-glass opacities with a predominantly lower lung zone distribution. This pattern, along with the presence of macrophages on bronchoalveolar lavage, is characteristic of DIP and helps differentiate it from other interstitial lung diseases.

Treatment/Management:

The management of Desquamative Interstitial Pneumonia (DIP) primarily focuses on smoking cessation and avoidance of environmental triggers. In individuals who continue to smoke, disease progression is likely. Supplemental oxygen therapy may be necessary in cases of hypoxemia.

Corticosteroids are often used as a treatment option, especially in individuals with progressive disease. Regular follow-up visits and monitoring of lung function are essential to assess disease progression and adjust treatment as needed.

The management of fundamentally involves instigating lifestyle changes that incorporate smoking cessation and the avoidance of specific environmental triggers that can exacerbate the condition.

This is of utmost importance as failure to quit smoking can cause the disease to progress further. In severe cases where a decrease in blood oxygen levels, referred to as hypoxemia, is observed, supplemental oxygen therapy is often recommended as part of the management strategy.

In addition, corticosteroids, known for their anti-inflammatory effects, are commonly employed as a treatment approach for DIP. They are particularly beneficial for patients showing signs of disease progression.

The regularity of follow-up visits, as well as continuous monitoring of lung function, is crucial in managing DIP. They not only provide an assessment of disease progression but also offer an opportunity to modify the treatment strategy as per the patient's evolving condition and needs.

Conclusion:

Desquamative Interstitial Pneumonia (DIP), a distinct form of interstitial lung disease, is primarily defined by the considerable accumulation of macrophages in the respiratory alveoli. While pinpointing the exact etiology continues to be a challenge for the medical community, it is widely agreed that factors such as smoking and exposure to certain environmental elements play a significant role in the disease's onset and progression.

Clinical manifestations associated with DIP can vary extensively, ranging from minimal discomfort to severe respiratory distress. Hence, reliance on clinical symptoms alone doesn't suffice for a concrete diagnosis, emphasising the importance of radiological evaluations. Tools such as chest X-rays and CT scans offer an in-depth perspective of the lungs' internal structure and help confirm the occurrence of DIP accurately.

As for management strategies, smoking cessation is an absolute requirement for halting disease progression, coupled with the avoidance of identified triggers.

Utilisation of corticosteroids can also be a part of the treatment approach, aiding in controlling the progression of DIP. Despite the challenges associated with DIP, it is important to recall that with early detection, accurate diagnosis and effective management strategies, the condition can be managed, ultimately enhancing the quality of life for those affected.

Desquamative Interstitial Pneumonia is a form of interstitial lung disease characterized by alveolar macrophage accumulation. While the exact etiology remains unknown, smoking and environmental factors play a significant role.

Clinical symptoms can vary, and radiological evaluation is crucial for accurate diagnosis. Smoking cessation and avoidance of triggers are essential in managing DIP, and corticosteroids may be used to control disease progression.

References:

1. Travis WD, et al. Desquamative interstitial pneumonia and respiratory bronchiolitis-associated interstitial lung disease. Seminars in Respiratory and Critical Care Medicine. 2008;29(6):641-657.
2. Vassallo R, et al. Smoking-related interstitial lung diseases. Clinics in Chest Medicine. 2012;33(1):165-178.
3. Churg A, et al. Desquamative interstitial pneumonia. American Journal of Surgical Pathology. 1990;14(6):526-535.